W9-BLF-688

DATE DUE

Drugs and Sports

Look for these and other books in the Lucent Overview Series:

Drugs and Sports

by Judith Galas

LUCENT
BOOKS

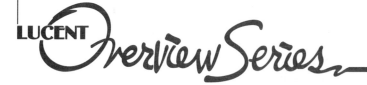

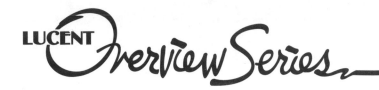

Library of Congress Cataloging-in-Publication Data

Galas, Judith C., 1946–
    Drugs and sports / by Judith Galas.
        p.   cm. — (Lucent overview series)
    Includes bibliographical references and index.
    Summary: Examines the issue of drug use by athletes, both to
enhance performance and as an escape, and includes a discussion
on drug testing.
    ISBN 1-56006-185-5 (alk. paper)
    1. Doping in sports—Juvenile literature.   [1. Doping in sports.
2. Athletes—Drug use.]   I. Title.   II. Series.
RC1230.G35   1997
362.29'08'8796—dc20   96-9854
                                                                              CIP
                                                                               AC

Contents

Introduction

"WINNING ISN'T EVERYTHING, it's the only thing." This often repeated comment of a famous National Football League coach, the late Vince Lombardi, captures an attitude held by many fans and athletes: sports is always about winning. This urge to win at all costs encourages the intrusion of drugs into sports. For if winning is everything, then many athletes will do anything to win. Sometimes doing anything means doing drugs.

The win-or-lose attitude not only limits people's view of sports, but it also misses an important part of athletic competition. Many athletes work hard to be the best they can be, not just to win. Personal growth also is an important part of sports, says Ronald Laura, former world power-lifting champion. Laura believes training and competition make the athlete a better person. "As long as the goal of sporting games presupposes that winning is in itself an ultimate value, the temptation will be to forsake *the value of being the best that one can be* in favor of simply being better than one's competitors."

Drug decisions

Whether they play in professional leagues, college and high school events, or Olympic and other world-level competitions, more and more athletes face a personal decision about drugs. Should they use drugs or should they stay clean?

Most athletes know that the path to gold medals, championships, scholarships, trophies, big paychecks, and Super Bowl rings often includes drugs. Those who stay clean

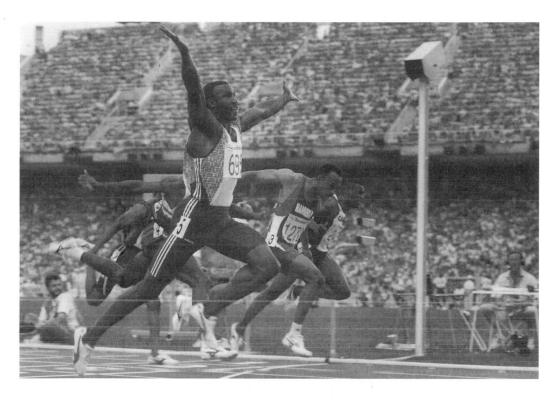

know they play against athletes who use drugs and thus may gain an unfair advantage. Some truly wish they did not feel pressured to use drugs. But like it or not, and regardless of what the truth may be, many believe that drugs are a part of winning or even surviving in sports.

In their book, *Drug Controversy in Sport*, champion Laura and former Australian rugby international star Saxon White ask an important question: "What is it about winning that makes it so important, even worth risking one's life for?" They note that the drug problem in sports may simply be a part of the drug problem in society at large.

Many people besides athletes, they say, want to take shortcuts to achieve their dreams. Many people want "maximum achievement with the minimum of effort." Laura and White write that people in general continually seek instant gratification. "In regard to drugs, we have been seduced by the power of the pill as if the medicine cabinet was an armory of magic bullets, to be used against the enemies of hard work and persistent effort."

Britain's Linford Christie sprints across the finish line to win fame and a gold medal in the 1992 Olympics. For some athletes, the desire to win at all costs results in the use of performance-enhancing drugs.

Early athletes used drugs

History, however, confirms that the use of chemical shortcuts to success in sports is an age-old problem. Recorded drug use goes back more than two thousand years. The Roman gladiators, who ate mushrooms and seeds that affected the mind, also drank herbal stimulants to dull their fear and to make them stronger and more able to withstand pain. The Aztecs used cactus-based stimulants that were like strychnine, a powerful rat poison. Stimulants also helped knights endure the jousts.

The slang word *dope* arose among ancient Africans. In the Kaffir dialect of southern Africa, *dop* referred to a stimulating liquor used by tribesmen in religious ceremonies. The Dutch discovered and used dop in the 1600s; later they spelled it dope. In the 1800s, dope came to be known as a mixture of opium and narcotics given to racehorses. In time, human racers used it as well. Today, dope refers not to any particular drug, but to drugs in general.

In 1865 swimmers in Amsterdam took dope, as did cyclists competing in Europe. Cyclists also drank *vin Mariani*,

Throughout history, athletes have relied on chemical substances to gain a competitive edge. Roman gladiators, for example, used drugs to help them withstand the pain and fear of combat.

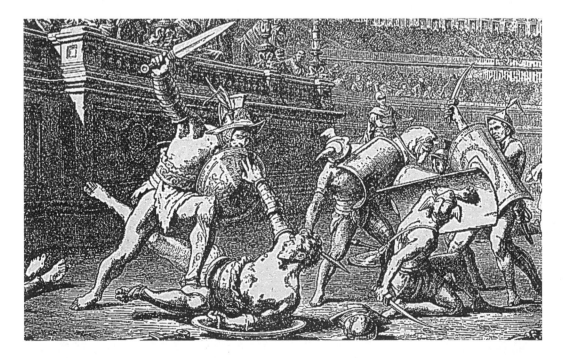

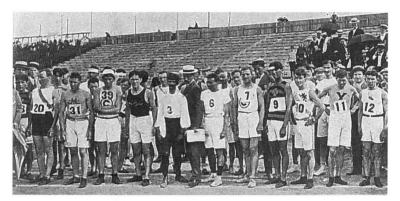

Marathon runners line up during the 1904 Olympics. Although Thomas Hick ultimately won the race, he risked his health—and even his life—by ingesting strychnine before the run.

also called "wine for athletes," a mixture of wine and an extract from the coca plant, which is the source of the addictive drug cocaine.

First recorded death of a cyclist

Cycling, a physically grueling sport, pushed many athletes of the late 1800s to use unusual means to prolong their endurance. Belgian cyclists took sugar tablets soaked in ether, the French took caffeine tablets, and the British inhaled pure oxygen. The first recorded drug-related death among cyclists occurred in 1866: an English cyclist died as a result of an overdose of a form of ether.

By the early 1900s, some athletes were lacing brandy with the poison strychnine. In small amounts the drug enhanced endurance and speed; in larger amounts it brought death. In 1904 Thomas Hick almost died after drinking the mixture before he ran (and won) the marathon at the Olympic Games in St. Louis.

Amphetamines became popular in the 1950s. Students used them for late nights of studying, long-distance drivers used them to stay awake on the road, dieters used them to promote weight loss, and athletes took them to increase their endurance and determination.

During the 1950s, most people basically saw drugs as useful. The drug research that grew out of World War II had brought many new drugs to the mass market. Vitamins and antibiotics, for example, helped people, pets, and livestock. This positive attitude about drugs is reflected in a

1958 report from the American College of Sports Medicine, which found that 35 percent of the 441 trainers, coaches, and assistants surveyed either had used amphetamines, known as "speed," or knew how to use them. Drug use, it seemed, was fairly widely accepted.

More cyclists die

In 1960 the Danish cyclist Knud Jensen died from stimulants at the Rome Olympics during the 175.38-kilometer road race. His trainer had given him a mixture of nicotinic acid and amphetamines, known as the "Knud Jensen diet." The combination of a hot Italian summer and a heart drugged to pump at top speed overpowered Jensen's body. At the same Olympics, 400-meter hurdler Dick Howard died from a heroin overdose.

Another heroin-related athlete death in 1965 prompted sports organizations in France and Belgium to push their governments to pass tough antidoping laws. But the death of British cyclist Tommy Simpson in 1967 reminded people that laws alone cannot keep athletes from using potentially dangerous drugs. The top cyclist of his day, Simpson had almost completed a six-thousand-foot climb in the heat when he collapsed into a coma and died. Rescuers found a vial of speed in his pocket; the substance was found in the corpse, as well.

A year later Jacques Anquetil, five-time winner of the prestigious bike race the Tour de France, gave up his trophy rather than take a urine test for drugs. "I dope myself," Anquetil said.

> Everyone . . . who is a competitive cyclist dopes himself. Those who claim they don't are liars. . . . Obviously we can do without them in a race, but then we will pedal fifteen miles an hour. Since we are constantly asked to go faster and to make even greater efforts, we are obliged to take stimulants.

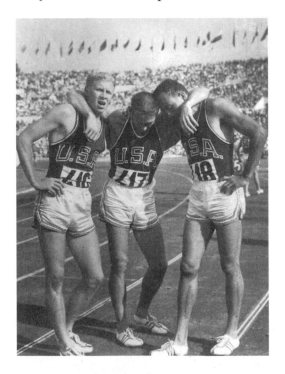

Hurdler Dick Howard (right) after the 400-meter race at the 1960 Olympics. Howard, who used heroin to enhance his strength and performance, later died from an overdose.

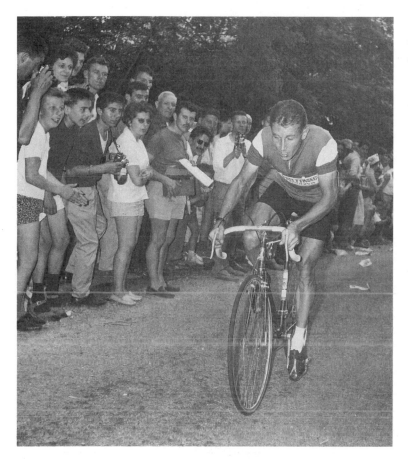

Cyclist Jacques Anquetil (pictured) publicly admitted that he and other cyclists used stimulants to counteract fatigue and increase alertness.

Between the 1950s and 1980s, athletes and sports fans knew that some athletes took and abused drugs, but not many people acknowledged the real impact of drugs on fair competition. Attitudes changed at the 1988 Olympics in Seoul, South Korea. These games marked a major turnaround in people's awareness and tolerance of drug abuse in the elite sports.

That summer the Bulgarian weight-lifting team left Seoul in disgrace. Two of its gold medalists—Mitko Grabley and Angel Guenchev—tested positive for the diuretic furosemide. The International Olympic Committee (IOC) disqualified the two men and revoked their medals. Hungarian weight lifter Andor Szanyi failed a drug test and returned his silver medal. Australia's Alex Watson, a pentathlete, or competitor in a five-event series, was

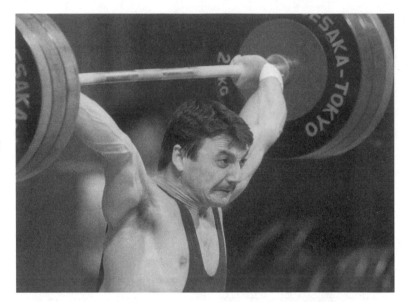

Grimacing under the weight of 160 kilograms, Angel Guenchev achieves a new world record at the 1988 Olympics in Seoul. Guenchev later tested positive for the diuretic furosemide and lost his gold medal.

expelled when his urine showed illegally high levels of caffeine. Then a Spanish pentathlete was expelled for drug use. By the end of the first week, ten athletes had been disqualified—about the same number as were expelled in 1984. But 1988 offered sports fans one final jolt. Canada's Ben Johnson, who had won the gold in the 100-meter dash, was disqualified because of drugs.

The 100-meter dash

Of all the events in the Summer Games, the 100-meter dash attracts a huge number of viewers. Even people who have little interest in track-and-field events often stop to watch this race. With its burst of speed, fleet athletes, and quick finish, the dash captures people's imaginations. So it is no surprise that an estimated seventy thousand people in the stands and more than two billion television viewers saw the race between Johnson and his arch rival Carl Lewis of the United States. If Johnson was going to beat Lewis, he would do it at this race.

Lewis had earned four gold medals in track and field in 1984, including one for the 100-meter dash. He had placed that gold medal in his father's casket and assured his mother that he would win another in 1988. So when the starting gun was fired, billions of people held their breaths—but not for long.

In a record-breaking 9.79 seconds, Johnson, not Lewis, crossed the finish first. He had run 328 feet, almost the length of three basketball courts, in about the time it takes to make ten loud finger snaps. He had beat second-place finisher Lewis by 0.13 second—practically the blink of an eye. Johnson was an instant hero; he was the fastest man on earth.

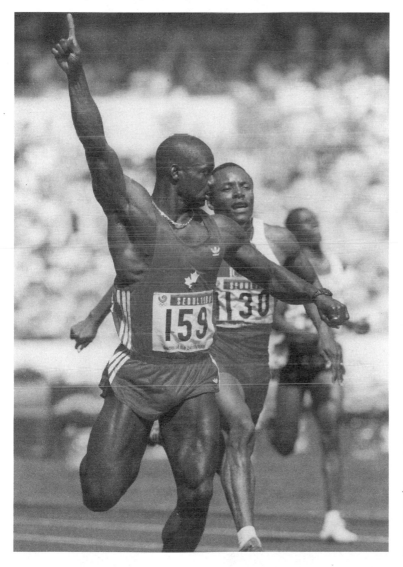

Ben Johnson sprints to victory during the 1988 Olympics. Johnson's fame as the fastest man alive lasted less than a day; he lost his gold medal after testing positive for steroids.

At the press conference following his win, Johnson said: "I'd like to say my name is Benjamin Sinclair Johnson, Jr., and this world record will last 50 years, maybe 100." It lasted less than a day.

Success to shame

The image of Johnson standing on the podium in victory quickly was replaced with photos of Johnson as he fled Seoul in disgrace, a briefcase shielding his face from photographers. Johnson had tested positive for steroids. He was stripped of his record and his gold medal.

Those who had been fighting for a cleaner Olympics saw a bright side to Johnson's shame. Johnson and his 100-meter dash, more than any single sporting event before or since, made the world face the problem of drugs and sports. Even before Seoul's Olympic torch was extinguished, the IOC, the various national Olympic committees, sports federations, and government panels were planning meetings, hearings, and investigations into drug use in amateur sports.

Many coaches, trainers, and athletes also were thinking about Johnson and drug use. But their thoughts were on ways of using drugs without getting caught. These are the members of the sports community who wonder why they should not use drugs when so many others do. The answers have to do with ideals, health, and fairness.

The sports ideal

The sports ideal is strongly linked to the belief in fair competition and personal sacrifice. The image of an athlete is of someone who works hard in the pursuit of excellence. Day in and day out, athletes push their bodies to excel. They watch what and how much they eat; sometimes they give up a personal life to devote themselves to achieving excellence in their sport.

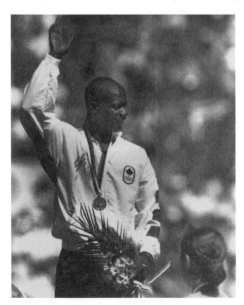

Ben Johnson waves to the crowds after receiving his gold medal. The Olympic committee later revoked Johnson's medal and he left Seoul in disgrace.

In the ideal, athletes also share a love of the game. Power lifter Laura sees this love as one of the essential and positive elements of sports. There's "a philosophy of sport which motivates play for its own sake—for the love of the game, if you like—and which sees sporting interaction as an activity which serves to enhance human integrity rather than just human performance."

But when drugs enter the sports arena, the idea of personal best or love of the game is replaced with personal deception and love of winning. An athlete no longer improves to win, but deceives to win. The loser may be a Carl Lewis, who trains hard without drugs, but loses to a Ben Johnson, who wins by a tiny margin because of drugs.

Those concerned about drugs in sports also worry about the impact on young people of the example set by drugged sports heroes. Athletes' lives seem to offer a message: if you work hard, focus on your dreams, and keep yourself clean and honest, you too will succeed. When top athletes are caught using drugs, their actions send other messages. First, it's OK to use drugs. Second, you can win only by cheating. Finally, not even the best athletes can win on their own merits.

The image of health and fitness

Top athletes who use drugs also negate the image of an athlete as someone who is physically fit and healthy. Since the first Olympics in Athens in 776 B.C., sports competitions have showcased the power and beauty of the human body. A beautiful body is healthy inside and out.

But drugs put an otherwise healthy body at risk for kidney and liver failure, cancers, heart and lung diseases, addictions, and depression. Even clean athletes face health risks from drug abuse. Drugs like anabolic steroids make people hostile. Players on these drugs can be overly aggressive, and in contact sports they may seriously injure other players.

Drug abuse among athletes is not just speculation. Some athletes at all levels of competition are abusing

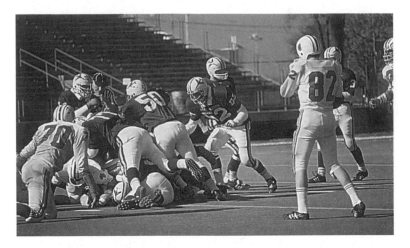

While no one really knows the extent of sports-related drug abuse, the problem affects athletes at many levels and in a variety of sports.

drugs. No surveys or studies can accurately assess the seriousness of the problem, for athletes, coaches, trainers, recruiters, and even parents of younger athletes are reluctant to admit drug use. But even coaches, owners, and universities—those who benefit from winning teams and famous athletes—know that drugs are bad for the sports image. As much as they may want their players to win, they do not want the bad publicity that comes when players are caught using drugs.

Others close to the problems of drugs and athletes say that drug concerns are exaggerated. Drugs—as needed and with professional supervision—have a place in sports, but drug abuse and self-experimentation do not. Many believe that athletes tend to overestimate the performance advantage some drugs can give. It is also suggested that other drugs do not in fact offer the desired benefits, which means that no unfair advantage results from taking them.

As common as drug use is, not all athletes use drugs. Many are clean, and they intend to stay that way. The athletes included in this book, for example, are not all drug users. But every athlete shown or mentioned in this book is affected by drugs in some way. If they are not taking drugs, they are competing against those who do. Clean or doped, every athlete will be tested time and time again for drugs. From this perspective, every athlete has a drug problem.

1

Athletes at Risk

IN THE WORLD of amateur and professional sports, illegal and legal drug use is all too common, says Robert Voy. As the former chief medical officer for the U.S. Olympic Committee (USOC), Voy saw a great deal of drug abuse firsthand.

If drug use and abuse is common, so are the risks. Athletes who take drugs to improve their performance and to cope with daily life face health problems ranging from depression and addiction to cancer and heart failure. They also run the risk of getting caught; athletes can be suspended from competition or even jailed. Drug use can damage reputations and finances, because many teams and advertisers shy away from players with drug problems. If using drugs is so risky, why do so many athletes take drugs?

NCAA survey

In 1985 and again in 1989 and 1993 the National Collegiate Athletic Association surveyed more than two thousand student athletes about their use of social and performance-enhancing drugs. The data from its most recent survey show that nationwide, eighteen- to twenty-five-year-olds are the people most likely to use illegal drugs. A large number of athletes fall within this age range, and many of them use drugs for the same reasons ascribed to millions of others: they take drugs to see what it's like, to relax, to have fun, to be cool, or just to fit in. But young athletes face some pressures the average young

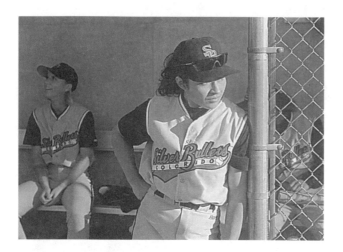

In the athletic community, the pressure to succeed can be great. Fear of failure and the desire to achieve excellence pushes some athletes to rely on chemical aids.

adult does not. They worry about their ability to be the best in stressful competitions, and they seek the high-dollar scholarships and contracts that go only to the best players. It is no surprise then that many are looking for the magic pill that will make them great. They want to run faster, pitch harder, pedal longer, and jump higher than the competition. They want to break records; they want to be famous; they want to be rich. Too often, drugs seem a reasonable way to satisfy those wants and to face the accompanying pressures.

Being the best

Few successful athletes are naturally athletic, but most are dedicated, determined, and driven. They spend years building their bodies and improving their skills. They suffer through painful injuries and rigorous workouts. Many give up a social life or move away from friends and family so they can focus on their training.

Naturally many worry that their bodies will not come through for them. They wonder whether drugs might give them that extra insurance. Some ask themselves, Should I take drugs and win or play fair and lose? Those asking that question are probably too insecure to stay clean.

The fear of failing can be so strong that even those who are punished for drug use find themselves reaching for the bottle or the syringe again. Sprinter Ben Johnson knew the cost of illegal drug use. His gold medal was stripped, he was suspended from competition for two years, and his liver was damaged from the steroids.

In 1989 a contrite Johnson spoke to the U.S. Congress: "I'm here to tell people that it's wrong to cheat. Don't take drugs. They're bad for your health. I was lucky: I got caught."

Four years later, Johnson's urine tested positive for unnaturally high levels of testosterone. This time the International Amateur Athletic Federation banned him from racing forever.

Sports agent Joe Douglas said Johnson probably could not face racing without drugs. "He has talent, but his performances are chemical," said Douglas. "All of a sudden there's attention, there's fame, there's money." Johnson may have feared that without drugs he would never see those rewards again.

Even after losing his gold medal and damaging his health, Ben Johnson continued to use chemical substances to enhance his performance. The International Amateur Athletic Federation has since banned Johnson from racing forever.

Money and fame

The lust for money and fame often drives the need or the desire for drugs. Young players want to land big pro contracts or scholarships to prestigious colleges. Professional athletes want to land lucrative deals with advertisers.

In a commentary for *Business Week*, Skip Rozin notes that sports have entered the "Age of Moneyball," with megacontracts and multi-million-dollar endorsements. "Sports seems to be sending the wrong message to young athletes striving for the deals that will set them up for life: It's O.K. to pop or inject steroids to enhance your performance."

Sometimes, however, drug use backfires. Instead of helping a young athlete make big money, the drug abuse is made public and ruins a player's reputation. After the 1988 Olympics, Johnson lost the opportunity to make about $30 million from endorsements and appearance fees.

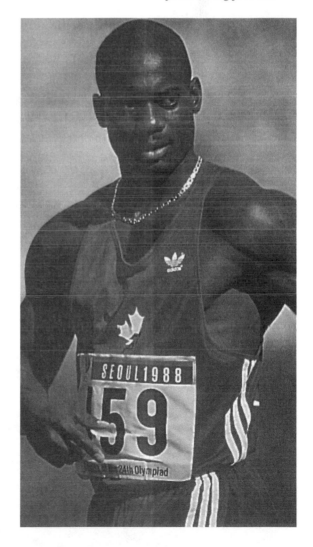

Drug stigma

Shot-putter Mike Stulze also learned this lesson. Stulze, twenty-three, a senior at Texas A&M University, won the Olympic gold in the shot put at the 1992 Summer Games in Barcelona, Spain. No American had won the shot put since 1968. The press and advertisers should have clamored for him. His best put at 71 feet, 2½ inches beat the silver medalist by 29 feet, ¼ inch—the biggest winning margin in the shot put since 1900.

But advertisers shunned Stulze. None of them wanted their products linked to an athlete who had already served a suspension for drugs. Although Stulze denied ever using steroids, tests in earlier meets had come up positive. The drug records of other shot-putters had also brought a stigma to the sport and to its winners. So when most manufacturers of athletic equipment were begging athletes to wear or use their products, Stulze had to buy his own shoes. In his case, drugs did not buy money and fame. "No one wants shot-putters," he said.

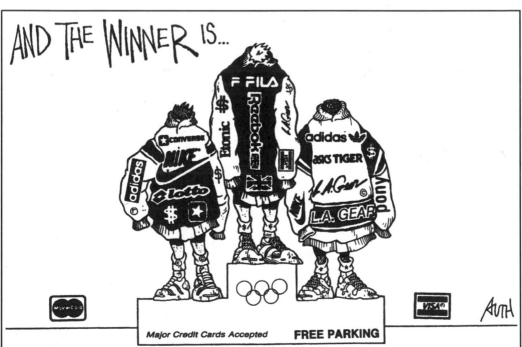

Self-esteem

In addition to the money and fame, many athletes also yearn for self-esteem. They want to feel good about themselves. Doing well on the court, course, or field is closely tied to how worthwhile they feel as individuals. The people who surround athletes each day are the very people who depend on them to perform well: coaches, trainers, owners, teammates. Most family members and friends who love them for themselves alone are miles away, perhaps in other countries.

Many athletes also are lonely. They have few, if any, friends outside sports. Many athletes also do not know how to just play: sports is their job; it is not relaxing. Given the loneliness, tension, and feelings of worthlessness, it is not surprising that many athletes turn to alcohol, cocaine, nicotine, or amphetamines as a way to have fun and feel good.

Outside pressures

Coaches, team owners, fans, parents, and peers indirectly or directly exert pressure on athletes to use drugs. Fans, for example, love their teams, but they can be hard on the players. They cheer them when they win, and curse them from the stands—often loudly—when they do not. They expect athletes to always perform well. The more popular an athlete becomes, the more pressure he or she is likely to feel from the fans.

Like fans, coaches want their players to always do well. Whether they coach at a university, in the pros, or for the Olympics, coaches are under pressure from team owners, alumni, or their country to produce a winning team or player. They pass this pressure along to the athletes. They may persuade an athlete to take drugs that will permit him or her to compete injured, or they may look the other way if they suspect players are taking drugs to improve their performance.

Drug cover-up

In fact, says Robert Voy, drug abuse is covered up by coaches and trainers, team doctors and owners, and national and international sports federations. These are the very people who should be stopping it, he says, but they also are the people who stake so much on the wins. "Many people at the USOC," the organization's former medical chief continues, "were in their business for one reason: to bring home the gold. Just how the athletes accomplished that—well, few really cared."

Professional cyclist Paul Kimmage learned firsthand that he was expected to use drugs if he wanted to ride. In 1990 Kimmage wrote a "tell-all" article on drugs for

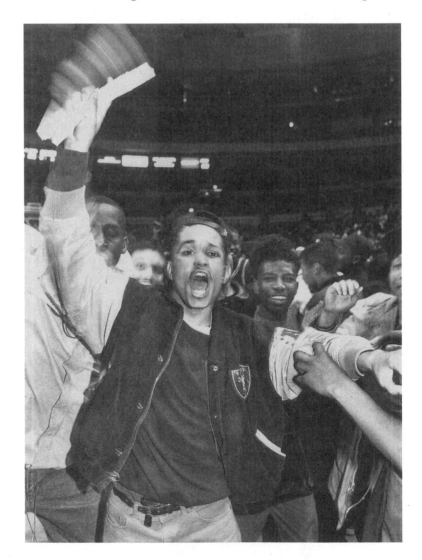

Athletes—especially those in the public spotlight—often face tremendous pressure from fans who want their players to perform well.

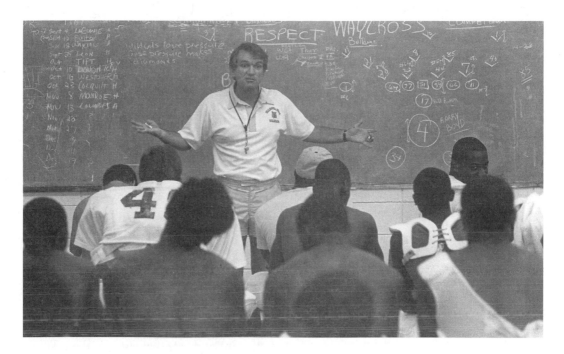

A high school football coach preps his players during a team meeting. The pressure to be the best often extends to coaches as well as athletes.

Bicycling magazine. A team rider on the professional cycling circuit, Kimmage described himself as a victim of a system that promoted drug use. He wrote:

> I was a sensible, strong-willed, good Catholic Irishman, and I would have sworn on any Bible that I'd never take illegal substances. I believed only cheaters took drugs, and I would never stoop that low. But when I entered the system, all that changed.

To stay in his bike saddle and compete professionally, Kimmage went from boosting himself with nothing more than a vitamin C drink, to letting the team caretaker legally inject him with vitamin B and iron. Then he let a teammate illegally inject him with amphetamines. "The next logical step for me was to hormones or steroids. It was a step that I was sorely tempted to take—but I never did. It had nothing to do with scruples or morals. No, it was simply the nature of the drug that scared me."

Family pressure

Pressure from parents also may result in drug use by young athletes. Some parents can almost taste the fame and fortune that comes to world-class athletes, so they want their child to be successful. Some parents send the message that they will love the child more if he or she wins, less if the child loses. Youngsters who feel that their parents' approval depends on a win may turn to drugs as a way to guarantee the love.

Bob Goldman, a world champion strength athlete who earned more than twenty world records, says he felt the link between winning and approval. Now a member of the Sports Medicine Committee of the Amateur Athletic Union, he is considered to be the leading authority on drug abuse in sports. An author of two highly regarded books— *Death in the Locker Room* and *Death in the Locker Room II*, Goldman recalls his sports competitions as empowering and exciting:

> Some of the most memorable moments of my life have been during the years of sacrifice, pain, and challenge that sports challenges provided. But the double-edged sword—that strong insatiable desire to win not only the competition, but also the approval and adulation of friends and family—can warp the beauty of the moment.

Jubilant teammates congratulate their pitcher after a no-hitter game. While the thrill of victory is exciting, some athletes crumble under the pressure to win and the high expectations others have of them.

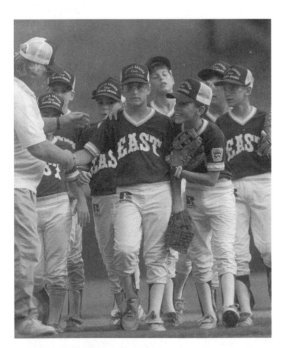

Team pressure

Teammates also pressure each other to use drugs. They may encourage the use of performance-enhancing drugs to make every member of the team fast and strong. Socially, they may promote alcohol, cocaine, and tobacco as a way for everyone to relax together or as a way for members to bond with each other.

Darryl Strawberry was a baseball player with the New York Mets when he became addicted to cocaine. "I didn't do coke until the majors in 1983," he says. In an interview with *Sports Illustrated*, he remembered a teammate coming up to him after a game to offer him some cocaine. "There's a couple of lines in the bathroom for you, kid," the older player said. "This is the big leagues. This is what you do in the big leagues. Go ahead. It's good for you."

Finally, the greatest source of pressure an athlete can feel can come from within. Former basketball star John Lucas, who is now a coach for the National Basketball Association (NBA), has been recovering from alcohol and drugs since 1986. In an interview for *Focus on Steroids*, Lucas told author Katherine Talmadge that the type of thinking that leads to drug addiction begins in grade school. "Sports can be an ego thing. You've got to be a winner. You want to be perfect."

When he played well he felt special; when he lost, he felt like a failure. Drugs made him feel less anxious about his playing. Today Lucas tells other recovering athletes that the uniform does not make the person. Today he says sports is what he does, it is not who he is.

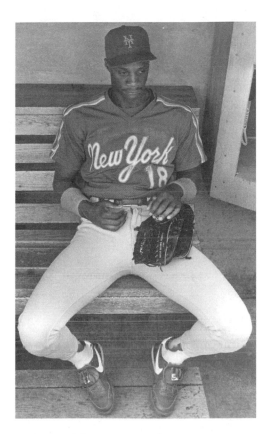

According to baseball star Darryl Strawberry, he became addicted to cocaine when teammates pressured him to use the drug for its energizing effects.

The media play a role

Former athletes Laura and White believe the media play a part in pressuring athletes to use drugs. The media help make superstars of talented young athletes, and these players naturally respond to the media's larger-than-life coverage of their achievements. They come to believe that their importance and self-worth rest entirely on their being able to win.

According to Laura and White, "Media attention can make or break an athlete." Before a big game or important competition, the media focus on an athlete's expected performance, introducing "a new dimension of pressure on an athlete apart from the pressure of the competition itself."

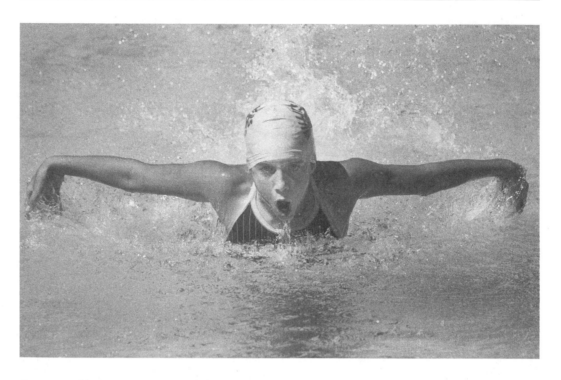

A young athlete competes in a swim competition. From high school to the pros, athletes may rely on drugs not only to gain an athletic advantage, but also to relieve stress and anxiety.

Athletes also want to look great and play extremely well for those watching in the stands or on television. Under the camera's bright lights, it's showtime. Athletes strive to do something extraordinary each and every time they're on. But it's unrealistic to assume that they will break a record every time they have the ball, dive into the pool, or race across the track. Drugs, however, make some of them believe they can.

Some reporters, so focused on the wins, also forget that sports is about more than winning. When China's young swimmer Liu Limin took the gold medal in the 100-meter butterfly in the World Student Games in Japan in 1995, the press hailed her success. Her win, they said, was a triumphant comeback for the Chinese, who had suffered setbacks from failed drug tests in 1994.

Three days later Liu missed the gold in the 200-meter butterfly by one-tenth of a second. Then the same reporters declared her loss a major setback for the Chinese. One-tenth of a second made the difference between being the comeback star to being a loser who had just embarrassed her country. When public honor or shame, success or failure rides on a fraction of a second, the pressure to get help from drugs can be enormous.

Easy success

In his commentary for *Business Week*, Skip Rozin saw one more reason for some athletes to use drugs—laziness. Less conditioned athletes can get an unfair boost from drugs. Rozin shared an observation by Harrison Pope, a psychiatrist at the Harvard Medical School:

> An athlete who is lackadaisical, who eats badly, sleeps badly, misses many days at the gym, works out without too much effort and takes steroids can blow away an athlete who works out to the limits of his ability, sleeps perfectly, has a perfect diet, and in every other respect goes to the limit of his body.

It is not unusual for people to want to succeed the easy way. It is also not uncommon for adolescents to want immediate results from any effort: they want to excel now, they want to feel good now. Young athletes tend to play down or ignore any advice that someday drugs may harm their health or their reputations. They see their bodies as machines they can control—take a pill and the body runs faster; get a shot and muscles bulk up; drink or smoke something and the body relaxes; pop a pill and the body sleeps.

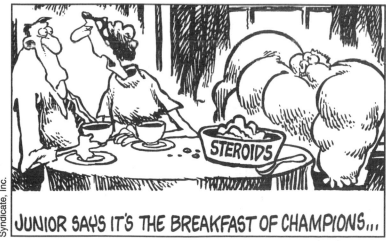

JUNIOR SAYS IT'S THE BREAKFAST OF CHAMPIONS...

For athletes who are stressed out, in pain, and struggling for success, drugs may make it easier to excel. For those who lack confidence in their abilities or doubt the love and respect of family and friends, drugs can make them feel good temporarily. For those seeking money and fame, drugs seem to offer some reassurance of success. With so much at stake, many athletes stake their future on drugs.

2

Steroids

CITIUS, ALTIUS, FORTIUS. The Olympic motto calls
for athletes to be faster, higher, stronger. In the ideal, athletes can run faster, jump higher, and grow stronger because they practice long and hard, eat and sleep well, take
care of their bodies, and listen to their coaches. But life
does not always meet the ideal. Too often steroids, or
chemical body boosters, illegally contribute to an athlete's
strength and success. Two types of steroids affect athletes:
corticosteroids and anabolic androgenic steroids.

Corticosteroids

Corticosteroids come from substances secreted by the
adrenal glands, located near or on the kidneys. When
rubbed on the skin, corticosteroid drugs reduce acne and
allergic skin reactions. When injected into a joint, they relieve inflammation and pain from injuries. When inhaled,
they relieve asthma. So, athletes often have legitimate uses
for them.

To make sure these drugs are used legally, sports governing bodies monitor their use carefully. Corticosteroids
cannot be taken by mouth or injected directly into the
bloodstream or muscles. In this country, doctors are required to advise the NCAA, or the USOC and the IOC,
when athletes under their care will be taking these drugs.

Anabolic androgenic steroids

Those troubled by steroid abuse are especially concerned about anabolic androgenic steroids, the synthetic, or man-made, forms of the male hormone testosterone. These drugs, often called AAS, anabolic steroids, or just steroids, are the most controversial drugs in sports. *Anabolic* refers to the ability of the drugs to build up the body's muscles. *Androgenic* refers to the masculinizing effects that result from their use. These drugs can be taken as a pill or as an injection.

Many athletes, doctors, and trainers believe AAS increase the body's lean muscle mass and strength. Not all researchers agree, however. Some question whether steroids build the body any faster than simple weight resistance training. They question whether high doses are any more effective than low doses and whether the gains are really as dramatic as some users claim.

Many athletes, however, seem to be convinced that steroids offer a route to increased overall strength. So it is no surprise that steroids are used in sports where increases in power, endurance, and speed benefit the athlete. Heavy

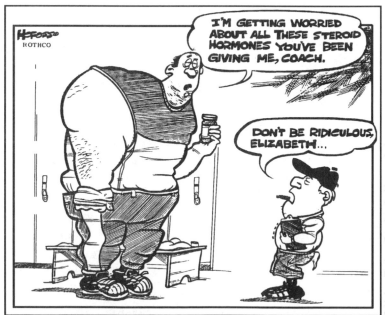

steroid users tend to be found among athletes in weight-lifting and track-and-field events, for example. Competitors in table tennis, women's field hockey, figure skating, equestrian events, and women's gymnastics most likely do not use steroids.

Unlike corticosteroids, the anabolic androgenic variety have few legitimate medical uses. Mostly physicians prescribe AAS to help men who have subnormal levels of testosterone or other hormone problems. Some researchers are using steroids to strengthen the bodies of those wasting away from AIDS. Most athletes, however, do not have a legitimate medical reason for using steroids, and their use without a prescription has been illegal in the United States since 1990.

Steroids in the 1950s

Athletes began using steroids in the 1950s, when they were still legal. John B. Ziegler, an American doctor on the medical staff of the 1956 World Games, saw athletes from the Soviet Union inject themselves with pure testosterone. The testosterone built up the muscles. But Ziegler saw that it also caused hair loss, shrinkage of the testicles, and enlargement of the prostate, a gland located near the bladder in men.

When he returned from Moscow, Ziegler helped develop Dianabol, known as D-bol. He wanted American athletes to have an athletic advantage without the side effects of straight testosterone. Ziegler had hoped to create a steroid that would build muscles without affecting masculine characteristics like body hair and voice pitch. But so far no one has developed a steroid that works on muscles only.

In the late 1950s, bodybuilders and weight lifters quickly adopted Dianabol. They saw that the combination of high doses of steroids and a strenuous regime of weight lifting increased their muscle size and body weight. It also increased their appetites and made them feel more powerful.

The recommended dosage was five milligrams, taken one to three times a day. But Ziegler found athletes using ten or twenty times this dose. Ziegler said he soon realized that he had created a monster and that he regretted his contribution to drug abuse in sports.

In the 1960s this steroid monster played a role in the cold war. Democratic countries like the United States and communist countries like those in Eastern Europe took their quarrels to the Olympics. Athletic skill became one way to measure political superiority. Anabolic steroids became the nonmilitary weapons of choice, and steroid use jumped sharply.

The 1964 Olympics probably were the first to see steroid use, with teams from the Soviet Union and Eastern Europe suspected of the most abuses. By the 1976 Summer Games in Montreal, steroid use was widespread. The IOC's drug-testing program included anabolic steroids for the first time that year—and some thought none too soon. The head of the East German swim delegation to the Montreal Games was asked about the deep voices of his women swimmers. His often reported reply was, "We have come here to swim, not to sing."

Illegal drug trade

By the mid-1980s, athletes from the West were going to the established steroid labs of Eastern Europe to buy drugs. Four Canadian weight lifters were caught in the Montreal airport with 22,515 capsules of anabolic androgenic steroids and 414 vials of testosterone bought in Eastern Europe. Ben Johnson's doctor, Jaime Astaphan, told Canada's Commission of Inquiry that he had obtained his steroids from the East Germans.

The illegal drug trade in steroids continues strong today. According to estimates from an international conference on steroids held in Prague, Czechoslovakia, in 1992 the yearly illegal steroid market in the United States alone stood at $500 million. Most of these illegal steroids are smuggled in from Europe and Mexico, with smaller amounts coming from South America and Asia. In a *Scientific American* story, writers John Hoberman and Charles Yesalis note that worldwide, the illegal sale and

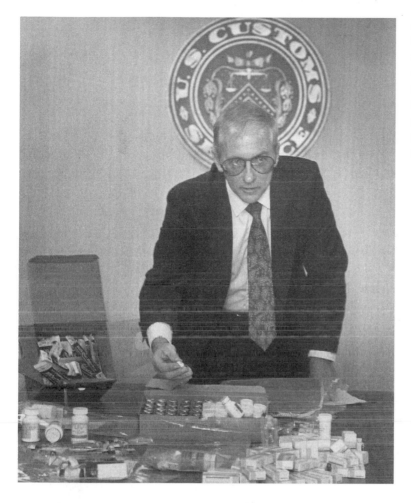

Each year, thousands of illegal drugs are smuggled into the United States. Here, a U.S. customs agent displays steroids seized during a nationwide campaign to combat the illegal drug trade.

use of steroids has "maintained a $1-billion international black market."

In the United States, steroid use without a prescription is prohibited by state, amateur, and professional athletic organizations, including the USOC and the NCAA. In 1994, however, the National Football League was the only professional sports program that randomly tested for steroids. The other professional sports clubs prohibit steroids but do not randomly test for their use.

In 1990 the U.S. Department of Justice classed anabolic steroids as a "controlled substance." This classification makes the nonprescription sale, use, or even possession of steroids a crime that can bring fines and jail time. The penalties, however, do not deter those determined to use steroids. "Federal officials spend thousands of hours each year prosecuting steroid cases, with little effect," says Skip Rozin, a commentator for *Business Week.* U.S. prosecutor Sean F. O'Shea told Rozin, "The public just doesn't perceive the dangers of steroids."

Health dangers

Many athletes shrug off the dangers. They have confidence in their health; their heart, lungs, muscles, and bones are at peak strength. "Die young, die strong, Dianabol" is a lighthearted chant among bodybuilders. The battle cry of some college football players was "Bury me massive!" Athletes think their bodies will tolerate the chemicals, even in unusually high doses.

Achim Albrecht of Germany flexes his incredible muscles after winning the Mr. Universe title in 1990. Steroid use appears to be particularly prevalent among bodybuilders and weight lifters because the drug increases muscle size and body weight.

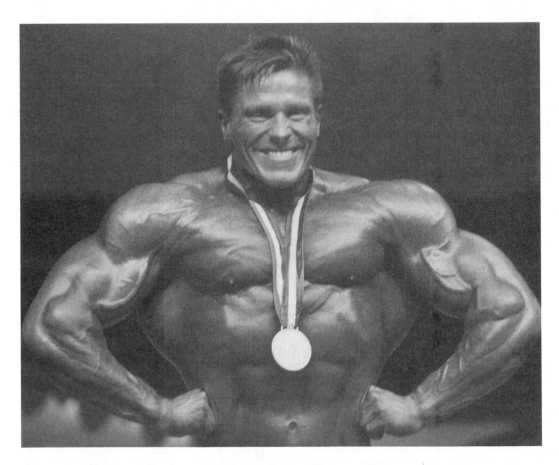

THE CONSEQUENCES OF STEROID USE

Below is a listing of the various health problems and conditions caused by steroid use. These consequences have been grouped according to gender.

In males

▶ impotence

▶ breast enlargement

▶ sterility

▶ shrinking of the testicles

▶ enlargement of the prostate gland, which can lead to difficulty urinating

In females

▶ irreversible male-pattern baldness

▶ irreversible lowering of the voice

▶ menstrual irregularities

▶ decreased breast size

▶ irreversible and excessive hair growth on body

To gain a competitive edge, some athletes routinely exceed the recommended dose of prescribed steroids, and most athletes quickly experience side effects. Many get acne. Male athletes have enlarged breasts and higher voices. Women grow facial hair and their voices become deeper. These changes may seem to be annoying or embarrassing rather than harmful. But athletes who use steroids regularly face more lethal problems.

Liver cancer, for example, is a common side effect of long-term steroid abuse. Anabolic steroids are broken down and cleaned out of the body through the liver, one of the organs that handles the body's waste products. Steroids also harm the kidneys, weaken the heart, and damage the circulatory system. Steve Courson, who played offensive guard for the Tampa Bay Buccaneers in the 1980s, used steroids. In 1989, when explaining to a reporter why he needed a heart transplant, he cited the drugs.

Measured against the quick benefits of strength, speed, and endurance, steroid dangers seem so remote. Athletes, says L. Scott Frazier at the Institute of Human Studies in

Aggression and hostility are common side effects of steroid use. Some athletes, however, believe these side effects are beneficial in sports such as football.

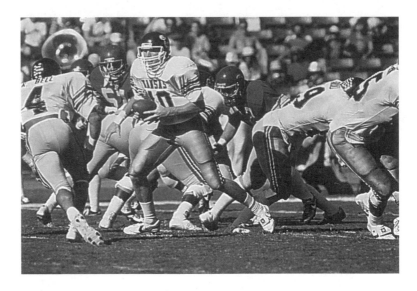

Sherman Oaks, California, do not want to hear bad news about steroids:

> They find it hard to think about the possibilities of life in their thirties or forties with damaged livers, premature baldness and . . . [mental] disorders. People want results. Results is why people are casting a blind eye to steroid abuse.

Emotional harm

As Frazier notes, steroids can harm not only the body, but also the mind. "Athletes on steroids," he continues, "become tense, nervous, irritable, highly aggressive, combative, seemingly [unaffected by] pain, self-destructive and suicidal." Intense aggression, often called a "roid rage," is a common side effect.

"Your whole mentality changes," says Joe, a young man interviewed for *Maclean's* magazine. "You go from an intelligent, normal guy to someone who resorts to beating people up if they don't agree with you. It's a totally physical mentality, and very aggressive."

Some athletes see these rages as a plus; for in addition to wanting strength and speed, some athletes want to be aggressive. Soccer and football players, for example, believe anger, impatience, and rage give them a valuable playing edge.

Some steroid users also become emotionally dependent on the drugs. They respond to their growing muscles in the same way a young woman with an eating disorder responds to her shrinking body. While the starving young woman looks in the mirror and is certain she is too fat, a young man on steroids looks in the mirror and sees a body that is too small.

In spite of all the known physical and emotional dangers, athletes continue to take steroids. In 1988 Dr. Forest Tenant estimated that as many as a million U.S. athletes were using anabolic steroids. Those high figures do not surprise most people in sports.

Steroid use soaring

In their 1991 book, *Drug Controversy in Sport*, Ronald Laura and Saxon White note, "The number of top-level athletes caught in possession of anabolic steroids has in recent years also soared, despite the introduction of legal penalties." In *Dying to Win: The Athlete's Guide to Safe and Unsafe Drugs in Sports*, author Michael Asken notes that almost 100 percent of competitive weight lifters and shot-putters rely on ability and steroids to win.

Widespread steroid use is not limited to men. The study on substance use and abuse habits among college athletes released by the NCAA in 1993 notes that steroid use in female college athletes in basketball, softball, tennis, and track and field showed considerable increases between 1985 and 1993. Increases were strongest in tennis and softball, with swimming showing declines in steroid use.

Like their male counterparts, female athletes are increasingly turning to steroids to gain an athletic advantage. A 1993 study indicates that steroid use among women increased between 1985 and 1993.

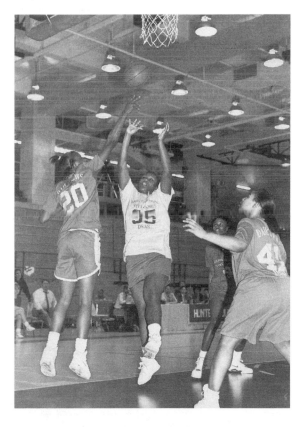

Wildor Hollmann, president of the World Federation of Sport Medicine in Cologne, Germany, said he saw the strong presence of steroids in women's sports. "I believe that today there are few women's world records in running, high jump, broad jump, shot put, discus and possibly javelin that have come about without the help of anabolic steroids," he said.

Some insist that steroid use is necessary in competition. Astaphan, who gave an anabolic steroid linked to liver cancer to Johnson, defended his actions before a drug investigation committee. "If you don't take it, you won't make it," he said.

Heart transplant candidate Steve Courson, the former NFL guard, had this to say in *Sports Illustrated*:

> The strongest people—the strongest athletes—in the world are all using steroids. They're being used not only in the strength field, but also in track and field and swimming. So you've got to be on drugs if you want to survive.

Youth and steroids

While many acknowledge and accept the widespread use of steroids by adult athletes, there is alarm over studies showing that steroid use is growing among young adults. A 1992 study in Oregon found that steroid use by high school football players had increased by almost 6 percent in two years.

In 1988 researchers at Pennsylvania State University concluded that thousands of teenagers may face steroid health dangers. The researchers studied 3,400 senior boys at 46 U.S. high schools and found that 6.6 percent had taken steroids. Using those figures, they estimated that 250,000 to 500,000 teens are taking or have taken steroids. About two-thirds started before they were sixteen years old. Those who took heavy doses for sixty to ninety days can expect to die in their thirties and forties, the researchers said.

In the 1990s the National Youth Sports Coaches Association surveyed more than 1,200 athletes between the ages of ten and fourteen: 2 percent said they were on steroids, 4 percent had been offered steroids, and 12 percent knew where to get them. Almost half thought steroids would help improve their athletic performance, and 43 percent incorrectly believed that steroids were not harmful if used properly. The latter response illustrated a common misconception, for there is no legitimate prescription use for anabolic androgenic steroids in young people.

Among NCAA Division I athletes, a 1991 study found a rise in use, with 16 percent of the men and 6 percent of the women saying they used steroids. Many researchers feel these numbers are too low. College athletes, they say, know steroid use is illegal and violates a long-standing belief in fair play. In embarrassment or guilt, these athletes are likely to underreport their use.

Youth at risk

Although steroids can harm anyone who abuses them, young athletes, whose bodies are still growing, are especially at risk. For example, steroids make a teen's natural hormone imbalances even worse; and when they cause the growth sites on the long bones to shut down, a teenage user's growth may be permanently stunted. Steroids can also make young athletes sterile—unable to have children.

Even though nonprescription steroid use is illegal and harmful, young athletes find ways to get the drugs. On

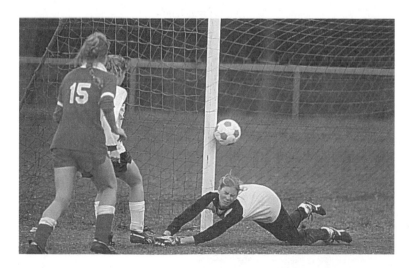

Young athletes are particularly vulnerable to the harmful side effects of steroids.

November 8, 1995, a report that four football players at Northwest Missouri State University had been arrested for buying steroids was aired on a news broadcast on KCTV-5 in Kansas City, Missouri. Two of the players had tested positive for the drug. The sales were reportedly linked to a seller known to be active in the Midwest.

The television reporter spoke with Frank Uryasz, director of sports science at the NCAA. Uryasz said the NCAA has been tracking anabolic steroid use among college athletes since 1985. Use has risen and fallen at various times. "It's not going down as much as we would like," he said. "Football is still the sport of highest risk for steroid use, but no sport is immune."

During the broadcast, Uryasz noted that illegal drug use is estimated to be higher among junior college athletes. Unlike the NCAA, the National Junior College Athletic Association has no mandatory drug-testing rules for college athletics. Junior colleges set their own testing policies, and drug use tends to be higher at schools without mandatory testing programs.

Role of education

Uryasz said he believes education plays an important role in reducing steroid use. The need to educate others about the danger of these drugs is what prompted Bob Goldman to write *Death in the Locker Room*. In that now famous book, Goldman mentions John, a young football star, who died from a rare form of kidney cancer brought on by steroids. John watched his diet. He did not drink, smoke, or stay up late; but he took anabolic steroids before their dangers were generally known. Like many people involved with sports in the 1970s, Goldman had not worried about steroids. But John's death prompted him to research these drugs. Here is his conclusion:

> Now that I've finished my research, I'm no longer open-minded. I can state unequivocally that drugs, especially anabolic steroids, have no business in sports. Anabolic steroids bestow few benefits, and none worth the terrible risks of taking them.

3

Performance- and Appearance-Altering Drugs

AT THE MENTION of performance- and appearance-altering drugs, also known as PAAs, most people think only of steroids. While steroids are widely used within sports, they are only one type of illegal or banned PAA drug. Illegal PAAs include sex hormones and human growth hormones, and more addictive and dangerous drugs like amphetamines. All PAAs change the way an athlete looks or performs.

Sex hormones

Both the male hormone testosterone and the female hormone progesterone change the way an athlete looks and performs, but in different ways. Testosterone is taken by athletes like weight lifters and sprinters who want to build body size and strength. Progesterone, however, is taken by female gymnasts who want to keep their bodies small and childlike.

Testosterone is produced by the testes, the male reproductive glands. Like steroids, testosterone causes the body to build muscle and to develop masculine characteristics.

Testosterone abuse is a little harder to detect in drug tests. Until 1981 no test could detect unnaturally high levels of testosterone. Because the hormone occurs naturally in the body, athletes feel that even with the improved tests,

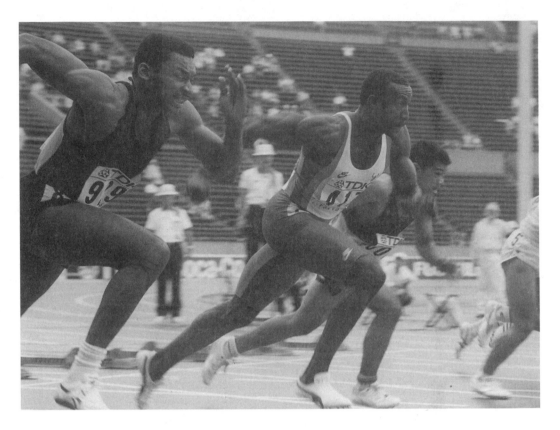

Linford Christie (right) starts the first round of a 100-meter race. While Christie's success is due to strenuous training, other athletes maintain that such physically demanding sports push them to use drugs.

they have a chance of getting away with artificially increased levels of testosterone to enhance their performance.

Young gymnasts may be using progesterone to enhance performance. This hormone, which plays an important role in menstruation (a woman's "period," or monthly bleeding), is made in the female ovaries, the almond-sized glands that contain the eggs from which human life may begin. High levels of progesterone stop menstruation and postpone the maturation of the body into womanhood. Some sports observers believe that female gymnasts are taking progesterone to stop their periods and to delay the time when they will have women's bodies.

"Brake" drugs

When used to hold off physical maturity, progesterone and similar hormones are called "brake" drugs because they halt or brake the body's development. Young girls on progesterone do not develop breasts or hips, which interfere with gymnastic performance by bringing about a shift in balance and a different response to gravity. For gymnasts who have been training since early childhood, putting off adult changes to their bodies gives them a few more years to compete. In *Death in the Locker Room II*, Goldman wrote:

> Many gymnastics watchers believe that the Eastern Europeans are experimenting with various [brake] drugs at the training camps they run for young athletes. . . . [M]any people are convinced that there is no way the Eastern European gymnasts can remain immature at eighteen and nineteen years of age without some kind of chemical interference.

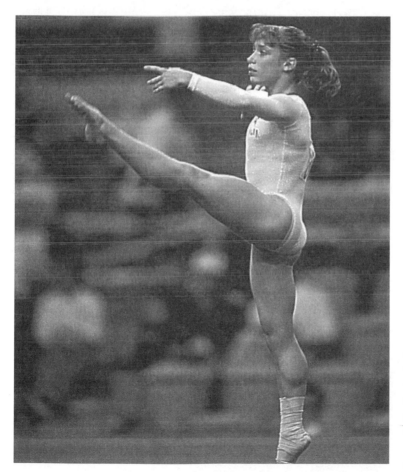

Gymnasts with small, physically immature bodies have an advantage over those who are more developed, prompting concern about the use of "brake" drugs in the gymnastic community.

Human growth hormone

Like sex hormones, human growth hormone (HGH) is a nonsteroid PAA. Athletes who take HGH injections believe that the hormone will work like a steroid to build muscle strength and to help the body recover more quickly after workouts. HGH occurs naturally in the body. It is secreted by the pituitary, or growth-regulating gland, which is located at the base of the brain.

Because HGH is found in everyone, it is hard to determine through drug tests whether an athlete has injected HGH. The hormone is on the International Olympic Committee's list of banned drugs. "But," writes Julie Cart in *Women's Sports and Fitness*, "officials admit [HGH] is nearly undetectable." Even endocrinologists, doctors who specialize in hormones, say "they are unable to tell when an athlete has taken HGH on her own or when her pituitary has secreted it."

At the inquiry into the illegal use of drugs at the 1988 Olympics, Jaime Astaphan admitted that he had prescribed HGH to the leading Canadian woman sprinter and had acquired fourteen bottles of HGH for Charlie Francis, the coach of most of Canada's sprinters.

Natural or synthetic, HGH is expensive; so only the wealthier athletes can afford it. In spite of its cost, the drug is becoming more popular. No research, however, clearly shows that HGH increases either strength or endurance. What the research clearly shows are the dangers.

Acromegaly

HGH causes distortions in body size as well as in appearance. Children whose bodies produce too much HGH grow into giants. After the teen years, a person with too much HGH develops acromegaly, a disorder of the pituitary gland.

"Acromegaly is beginning to be noted in athletes," says Bob Goldman of the Amateur Athletic Union. These athletes have "increased coarsening of facial features, increased size of the nose, lips, tongue . . . an underbite . . . with enlargement of the . . . jaw. The forehead becomes

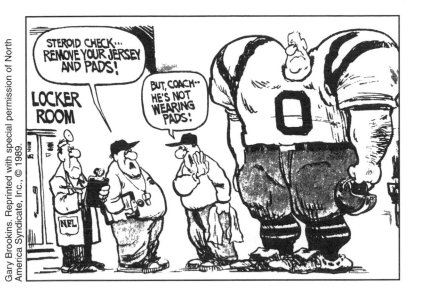

more prominent . . . and the fingers and toes widen into a spade-like shape." Increased sweating, skin discoloration, joint pain, congestive heart failure, and a risk of diabetes also can occur.

"Athletic acromegaly and selective gigantism is something we will begin to see more of," Goldman predicts. He continues:

> Unfortunately athletes tend to believe what is written in underground drug literature or other nonscientific sources. One individual who sells HGH to athletes wrote in a body building magazine that athletes who take this drug can "put on 40 pounds of muscle, with no change in waist size, and that they would increase in height. . . ." Well, needless to say they came from all over to visit this man.

Like HGH, the promises of a fairly new hormone-related drug known as EPO is attracting athletes' attention. Cyclists are especially attracted to this performance-enhancing drug, which is made from naturally occurring hormones. EPO is said to increase endurance by boosting the body's production of red blood cells, which carry oxygen throughout the body.

EPO is almost impossible to detect in drug tests because it disappears from the body within a few hours. But the drug thickens the blood, which can cause clotting and heart attacks. Between 1988 and 1990, five Dutch cyclists, ranging in age from twenty to thirty-two, died of heart failure. All were physically fit. Some speculate that they had been taking EPO.

Clenbuterol

Like HGH and EPO, the drug clenbuterol is growing in popularity because it is difficult to detect and because athletes believe it works like a steroid. In December 1995 a report in *Medicine and Science in Sports and Exercise* said athletes were turning to clenbuterol, a drug most often used to put more lean meat on cattle. The drug helps athletes lose fat while they gain muscle, a physical change especially desired by weight lifters. The report also said use among U.S. athletes was increasing because the drug is not policed in the same way as steroids.

In *Women's Sports and Fitness*, Cart wrote that clenbuterol offers a "triple whammy": it "has . . . muscle-building properties, acts as a stimulant and increases lung capacity." This combination also appeals to sprinters and

Like many other sports, competitive swimming is physically grueling. Swimmers are among the athletes who resort to PAAs because these drugs offer the benefits of strength and endurance that such sports demand.

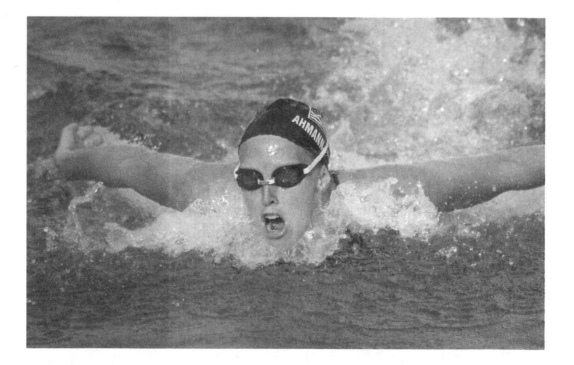

swimmers. Yet according to Irvine D. Prather of the University of North Texas Health Science Center in Fort Worth, who wrote the published report, the long-term effects of clenbuterol are unknown. In large doses it can give people muscle cramps and tremors, increase their heart rate, and make them tense.

Drugs like clenbuterol, testosterone, and HGH are more likely to be used by athletes who take steroids. The drug use survey released by the NCAA in 1993 found that while fewer college athletes were using PAAs, those who said they used steroids also used other PAAs. Among those who said they used steroids, about 20 percent also used testosterone, 11 percent used HGH, and 25 percent used clenbuterol.

Amphetamines

Like clenbuterol, amphetamines increase an athlete's heart rate and agitation, but they have been used for much longer than clenbuterol, and far more widely. Known on the street as bennies, dexies, goof balls, jolly beans, pep pills, uppers, or speed, amphetamines can be injected or swallowed as pills or capsules.

Amphetamines stimulate the brain and body. They temporarily boost self-esteem, increase physical activity, and make a person feel wide awake and excited. But they also can cause stomach ulcers, weight loss, skin disorders, brain damage, and diseases of the lungs, liver, kidneys, and heart. They can bring on stroke, heart failure, or lung collapse, cause mood swings, and make users nervous, depressed, unable to sleep, irritable, easily upset, and suspicious. They are also addictive; a person has to take more and more to feel good.

Amphetamines also may not really improve performance. Some studies suggest that rather than slowing the onset of fatigue, they prevent an athlete from feeling tired. Research also shows that improvements in performance may be obtained only in boring and repetitive jobs. Athletes taking amphetamines may not perform any better; they may simply feel that they are doing better.

Introduced in Germany in the late 1800s, amphetamines were first used by doctors to treat blood pressure, nasal congestion, some mental illnesses, and seasickness. By World War II, pep pills were freely given to soldiers. In the 1940s and 1950s, amphetamines turned up in sports, and athletes at all levels commonly took uppers. They were used heavily by Olympic athletes at the 1952 Winter Games in Oslo, Norway, where several speed skaters became ill from the drug. They were also popular with college athletes. One 1958 study revealed that one in four took speed.

Tightly controlled

Today the medical use of amphetamines is tightly controlled and is limited to treating some sleep disorders, hyperactivity in children, and obesity. Within sports, amphetamines have been regulated since the 1960 Rome Olympics. They are banned by all sports organizations, but remain popular with some athletes. Weight lifters, wrestlers, and jockeys who want to lose weight quickly before their events take amphetamines to speed up their metabolism. Skiers, speed skaters, and cyclists use the drugs to enhance their endurance.

"There are probably gold medal winners and world record holders from the United States who would never have even come near the winner's podium had it not been for their use of performance enhancing substances, and this is still happening," says former USOC medical officer Robert Voy.

Former professional cyclist Paul Kimmage did not compete in the Olympics and he does not hold a world record, but pro circuit cycling taught him to use speed. "It doesn't take long for the realities of pro cycling . . . to sink in. In my case, it took just 24 weeks to realize that cycling at this level was no longer a pleasurable sport, but rather a seedy business."

One day while preparing for a race, Kimmage felt a prick in his left shoulder. A teammate had injected him with amphetamines:

The effects were startling. Earlier I felt nervous, inferior and racked with self-doubt. But once the drug took hold, my character transformed. I felt a maddening urge to jump on my bike and ride all day. I was incredibly confident. I felt invincible. . . . Was I cheating? No, I was not. I was merely using the system. There was no dope control. If there had been, none of the riders would have used amphetamine. You see, in professional cycling the sin is not in taking drugs, it's in getting caught.

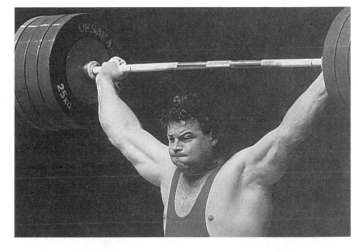

Training and competing can be intense psychologically as well as physically. Amphetamines stimulate both the body and the brain Users claim this type of drug makes them more alert, confident, and excited.

Easy to detect

Amphetamines are easy to detect through urine tests, so athletes at world-class competitions do not take speed before or during their events. In fact, a urine test can pick up a single dose taken as much as seven days before an event. Thus, regular testing at athletic competitions has led to better control.

Stimulant use is more likely at high school sporting events where testing for these substances is not done, and at some college competitions, since testing is not universal in contests at this level. In the study it released in 1993, the NCAA found that amphetamine use among college athletes had dropped. According to the self-reported figures, an average of 2.1 percent of those surveyed in 1993 had used amphetamines compared with 8.1 percent in 1985.

Almost 80 percent of those who said they did not use amphetamines said they had no need for them. Only about 5 percent said they did not use them because they were concerned about their health. Of those who did use amphetamines, more than 33 percent first tried them in high school and sixteen percent had done so in junior high or before.

Caffeine

Caffeine is a much weaker stimulant than amphetamines, but it probably is the world's most popular and widely available drug. Found in a variety of products such as coffee, tea, colas, cocoa, aspirin, and some cold remedies, caffeine is also used by athletes.

Caffeine stimulates the central nervous system, the heart, and the kidneys. It helps people stay awake, makes them feel more confident and positive, and at moderate levels can have a calming effect. Caffeine in concentrated doses—that is, at levels equal to thirty to forty cups of coffee—can, however, cause seizures and death.

Athletes such as cyclists and cross-country skiers use caffeine to increase their alertness and speed. Those who compete in archery and rifle shooting say they use caffeine to increase their concentration and to steady their nerves.

Athletes such as cyclists may rely on caffeine—the world's most popular drug—to boost alertness and speed.

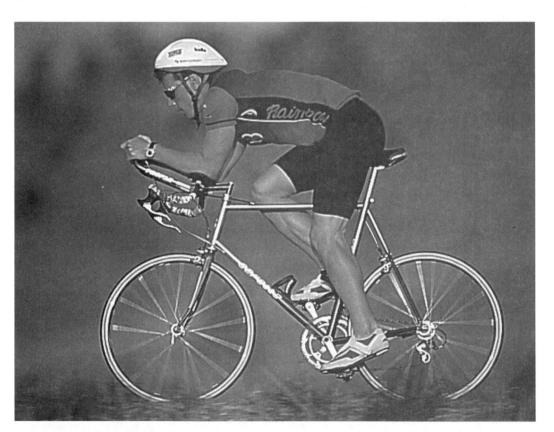

In the 1970s, one scientist recommended caffeine pills as a way to make the marathon "a fun run." Athletes of all ages started to pop caffeine tablets, and the IOC removed caffeine from its banned doping list, but just for awhile. Because high doses can affect the outcome of a competition, tests are done for caffeine, and it is easily detected by today's testing methods.

The IOC and USOC test for unusually high caffeine levels and suspend athletes who exceed the guidelines. Excessive levels can come from about six to eight cups of coffee taken three hours before testing. About ten cola drinks or several No-Doz tablets could also lead to a suspension.

L. Scott Frazier, of California's Institute of Human Studies, says that caffeine can be a mild, even a helpful stimulant. At large doses, however, it becomes addictive and harmful:

> After an athlete has relied on large doses of caffeine and wishes to stop, he or she may experience strong headaches accompanied by craving and depression. The depression may be long-lasting and can be complicated by tension, nervousness and irritability. . . . The disadvantages of caffeine-loading outweigh the benefits.

Getting PAAs

Most people assume that of all the PAAs, only caffeine is readily available to athletes. In fact, athletes can get even tightly controlled PAA drugs fairly easily. The National Federation of State High School Associations has a program for the prevention of alcohol, tobacco, and other drug use called TARGET, which has commented on athlete access to PAAs:

> Typically distribution of steroids and other illegal PAA drugs occurs in private gyms and fitness centers. [The drugs] are easy to access and usually pass from athlete to athlete, although coaches, agents, and doctors are sometimes involved. These PAA drugs are also marketed on the street through the channels used to distribute cocaine, heroin, and marijuana.

The TARGET report expressed concern that many athletes and their coaches believe that PAAs can help athletes in spite of all the research showing these drugs to be harmful and not helpful. "Many PAA drug users," it says, "make a distinction between their drug use behavior and that of individuals who use, for example, cocaine. They view their use of PAA drugs as behavior aimed at self-improvement, which is a valued societal goal."

Applause and adoration given to high-dollar athletes reinforce the idea that drugs bring rewards. It is such thinking that helps to give sports figures who use PAAs the mistaken impression that they are benefiting themselves and their sports.

4

Social Drugs

ATHLETES ARE RELUCTANT to admit their drug abuse and their addictions to alcohol, cocaine, marijuana, and nicotine. Coaches, trainers, parents, and recruiters also shrink from discussing drug problems. They do not want stories about drug abuse to damage the reputations of their professional clubs, Olympic teams, or high school and college programs.

Those who study drug abuse in U.S. sports think athletes' drug abuse reflects the general level of drug abuse found in this country. Drug use has gone up nationwide in the general population, so a rise can be assumed within sports as well.

Drug use is up

In its booklet, "Drugs and the Athlete . . . A Losing Combination," the National Collegiate Athletic Association (NCAA) notes that the government estimates that as many as 20 million Americans regularly use marijuana, and 500,000 abuse heroin. The National Institute on Drug Abuse estimates there are 5 million to 6 million cocaine users in the United States alone.

In her 1991 book, *Drugs and Sports*, Katherine Talmadge reports that one in ten teens has tried some form of cocaine, and the average age of a crack user is seventeen. There also are 10 million alcoholics in the United States, she says. More than 5 million teens have serious drinking problems, and half started drinking before the tenth grade.

In spite of higher drug use, people may be less concerned about the dangers of drug abuse. In January 1995, *Jet* magazine reported the findings of a federally funded study of youths. Lloyd D. Johnston, the head of the research team at the University of Michigan, attributed the increase in drug use among youth to a "glamorization of narcotics in movies and music." But Johnston's group also found that with the increase in drug use came a decrease in concerns about the health dangers linked with drugs.

In comparing its 1985, 1989, and 1993 surveys of drug use among more than two thousand student athletes, the

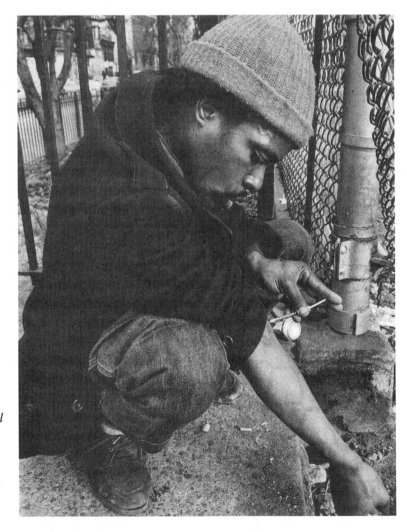

Drug use in the general population is on the rise nationwide. This man is among the estimated half million Americans who abuse heroin.

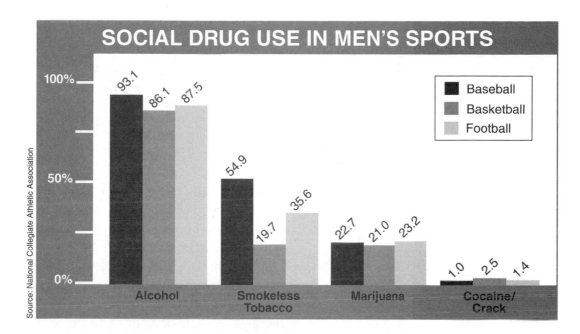

Source: National Collegiate Athletic Association

NCAA found that alcohol use remains high. The use of smokeless tobacco is growing, while the use of cocaine has dropped sharply. Marijuana, however, is still used by about one-quarter of the surveyed athletes.

Athletes who become accustomed to using drugs in high school and college most likely will continue to use drugs in professional sports. In the pros, the pressures are greater, and athletes have more money to spend on drugs.

Turning to social drugs

Athletes at all levels and in a variety of sports turn to so-called social drugs to alter the way they feel. These drugs help athletes relax or escape from the pressures. For a short time they can forget that they missed a free throw, dropped a pass, or struck out in full view of everyone. They can forget the high expectations others have of them.

"If I won, I went out drinking to celebrate," says Dwight Gooden, former pitcher with the New York Mets. "And if I lost, I went out drinking to forget about it."

In an article for *Student Assistance Journal*, drug educators Steven Milburn and Scott Smith note that athletes

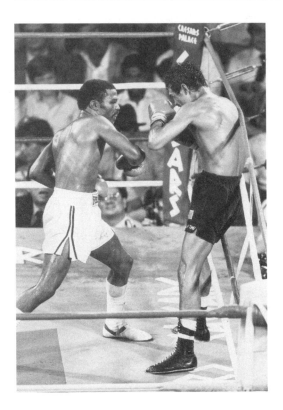

Boxing champ Aaron Pryor (left) releases a flurry of punches against his opponent. Pryor's life was ruined when he became addicted to crack cocaine.

probably use alcohol and other drugs for the same reasons they compete:

> The biochemical high an athlete gets from competition . . . is similar to the high he or she gets from alcohol and other drugs. Still pumped up from the adrenaline surge of competition, an athlete leaves the field needing to blow off steam.

Athletes, ill equipped to handle all the good or bad attention, can retreat into alcohol and other drugs to cope with the acclaim and criticisms. Once they become addicted to social drugs, however, they must cope not only with their addiction, but also with the damage to their personal and professional lives.

Aaron Pryor, a junior welterweight boxing champ, is still picking up the pieces from a life shattered by addiction to crack cocaine. Once a champion and a millionaire, Pryor has slept on the streets of Cincinnati and in prison. He has lost a mansion, cars, friends and family, his trophies, his reputation, and almost his life. He went from making millions as a fighter to working in the prison gym for 25 cents a day. In 1995, at the age of thirty-nine, he was out of prison, fighting to stay drug free, and earning $350 a week giving boxing lessons.

Cocaine

Pryor's addiction to crack and to powder cocaine and his story of struggle is not rare among athletes. In the 1970s, cocaine began to replace amphetamines as the most popular stimulant among professional athletes. Indeed, cocaine is the most popular drug in the sports world, says Mark S. Gold, founder of a national drug hot line.

Also known as coke, snow, blow, or flake, processed cocaine looks like powdered sugar or baby powder. It can be inhaled, swallowed, or injected. In general, users feel a rush right after taking this illegal drug. They may also feel mentally alert, upbeat, energetic and confident, and immune to pain. Some athletes—like football players—may take cocaine to feel more powerful and positive on the field and after a game.

In *Drugs and Sports*, Talmadge says some studies show that at least 20 percent of pro baseball and football players have used cocaine. Athletes themselves say the figure is much higher. Mike Strachan, formerly with the New Orleans Saints, was convicted of selling cocaine to other football players. Strachan estimates that 40 to 60 percent of all NFL players have used cocaine. Carl Eller, a recovering cocaine addict and an All-Pro defensive end with the Minnesota Vikings, agrees. He says about half of all pro football players have used cocaine, and one in five are addicts.

Crack is a cheap and broadly distributed by-product of cocaine. Looking like hard slivers of soap, crack is smoked and is even more addictive than powder cocaine.

Football player Mike Strachan talks to reporters after pleading guilty to drug charges. Strachan, who was convicted of selling cocaine, suggested that the use of cocaine is prevalent among NFL players.

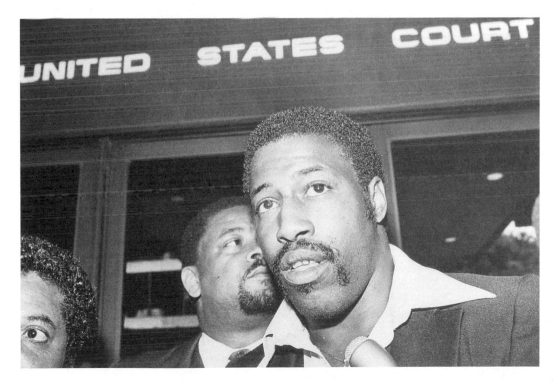

Crack gives the user a strong sense of pleasure and energy, but the high does not last long. When the drug's effects wear off, after about twenty minutes, people feel nervous, depressed, angry, and tired. As soon as they crash, they want to use the drug again.

Pros make headlines

Professional athletes linked to cocaine make the headlines. In March 1996, thirty-year-old Michael Irvin, all-time leading receiver for the Dallas Cowboys, was indicted on felony possession of at least four grams of cocaine. That same month a grand jury in Rockwall, Texas, indicted Pittsburgh Steelers running back Byron "Bam" Morris on felony drug charges. A leading rusher in Super Bowl XXX, Morris was twenty-four years old when he was indicted for possession of cocaine and marijuana.

In December 1992, John Lucas made headlines when the San Antonio Spurs hired him as the team's new coach. The job signaled the fourteen-year veteran's professional comeback after a long period of cocaine and alcohol addiction.

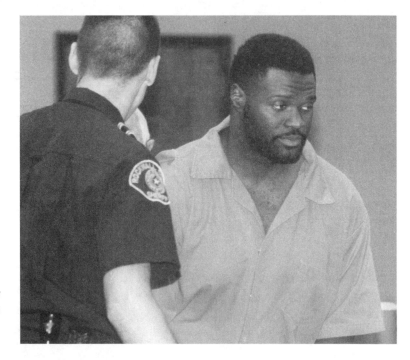

Pittsburgh Steelers running back Byron "Bam" Morris made headlines when he was indicted for possession of cocaine and marijuana.

Once considered to be one of the NBA's best point guards, Lucas had been fired by the Houston Rockets on March 13, 1986, as a result of testing positive for drugs in the wake of a coke binge. For almost a decade, he'd abused drugs and alcohol, despite four stays at a treatment center. His wife was said to have locked him in the house at night as a way to keep him off the streets and away from drugs.

Within days of being fired from the Houston team, Lucas entered his last drug treatment program. He recalls a drug counselor asking him to look into the mirror and tell what he saw. "I see a good looking black man," Lucas told the counselor. "The Number One pick in the NBA draft and one of the best point guards ever." The counselor responded, "I see a man who has lost his job for the third time and can't stay sober."

Young athletes and coke

Cocaine does not endanger only older, professional athletes like Lucas. It also affects college athletes. In 1991 Charles Thompson, a University of Oklahoma quarterback, was convicted of cocaine distribution after he tried to sell the drug to an FBI agent. He served seventeen months in a Texas prison and called the experience his "wake-up call."

In the 1985 NCAA survey of more than two thousand student athletes, 17 percent said they had used cocaine during the year. In the 1993 survey, the percentage had dropped to just over 1 percent. The 1 percent who used cocaine, however, reported more frequent use.

In all three reporting years, most athletes said they got their cocaine from relatives and friends. All said they used cocaine either to feel good or to be social. Almost half stopped using cocaine because they were concerned about their health.

Cocaine affects high school athletes, too. Of the college students who told the NCAA surveyors that they used cocaine, about 60 percent said they first tried the drug in high school. In his book, *Dying to Win*, Michael Asken

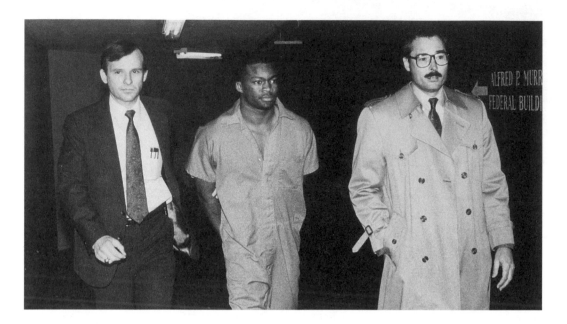

University of Oklahoma quarterback Charles Thompson jeopardized a promising football career when he became a cocaine dealer. Here, Thompson is led to court to face drug charges.

quotes a high school football player from South-Central Los Angeles. "You know how many people you run into who are dealing drugs? The ice cream truck goes by. I go out to buy a Popsicle and the driver says, 'I got a little more than ice cream here.'"

When they first begin using cocaine or alcohol, many athletes do not think about their health. They feel strong and invincible. They just want to see what it feels like to be high or drunk. They do not believe they will become addicted.

But cocaine in all its forms is highly addictive. It also causes headaches, nosebleeds, vomiting, sore throats, coughing, and sinus and muscle pain. It makes a player feel edgy, irritable, suspicious of others, and even suicidal. It can cause hallucinations, bring on sudden heart attacks, and damage the lungs and brain.

Alcohol dangers

Unlike cocaine, which stimulates the brain, alcohol slows it down. The American College of Sports Medicine has concluded that alcohol slows athletes' reaction time and disrupts their coordination, accuracy, and balance. Alcohol does not help an athlete's energy level, oxygen intake, or heart rate. It will not improve strength, endurance, or speed; over time, however, it will harm the heart, liver, brain, and muscles.

In spite of its potential harm, the consumption of alcohol is high in professional, college, and high school sports. Don Newcombe, a star pitcher for the Los Angeles Dodgers and a recovering alcoholic, says 10 to 15 percent of professional baseball players are alcoholics. Some think the figure may be as high as 35 percent.

"Alcohol is the drug most frequently used by athletes," says the NCAA. In its ongoing study of drug use among college students, the NCAA reports that alcohol use is high and remained almost unchanged between 1985 and 1993.

Almost 90 percent of the athletes surveyed said they drank alcohol. Almost half of those said they have six or more drinks each time they indulge. In 1993 almost 18 percent of the athletes who drank said they had their first drink in junior high and almost 63 percent took their first drink in high school. A survey conducted by the state of Minnesota showed that three out of every ten high school students use alcohol regularly.

Drug educators Milburn and Smith suggest that alcohol abuse among high school athletes may result from the coupling of alcohol and sports. Beer is sold at most athletic events, and ads for alcohol often are aired on television sports programs.

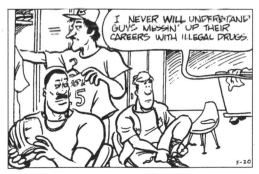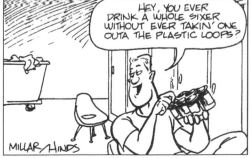

Alcohol claims more lives each year than anabolic androgenic steroids. But many coaches and researchers in sports medicine are more concerned about steroids than beer.

Two New York Mets

Players and managers with the New York Mets were not concerned about Darryl Strawberry and Dwight Gooden. Most everyone involved with the team knew that both star players drank heavily. But as long as the men did well on the field no one seemed to care much about their addiction. Each had been National League Rookie of the Year, Strawberry at twenty-one in 1983, and Gooden at nineteen a year later. By age twenty-five both men were baseball stars and millionaires. They played with the Mets when the team took the World Series in 1986. Strawberry, however, was too hung over to make the team's ticker-tape parade.

A hard drinker since 1986, Gooden admitted that he refrained from drinking only on the two nights before a Saturday starting assignment. At twenty-two he tested positive for cocaine and entered a drug rehabilitation program. At thirty he drank to avoid the emotional pain of facing his third straight losing season. "Drugs, alcohol . . . it's everywhere . . . you can never let your guard down," he says.

Gooden said that between 1986 and 1991, of the twenty-two Mets players who appeared in the 1986 World Series, eight were arrested for incidents related to alcohol, and a ninth was disciplined for cocaine.

Strawberry said he was drawn to the excitement of using alcohol and drugs:

> That's how I got addicted. It was an exciting way to escape from everything else. I came to the major leagues at such a young age, and coming to New York . . . maybe someplace else it would be a little different, but New York is a party place, an upbeat place.

Both men were treated at the Smithers Alcoholism and Treatment Center in New York City for drugs and alcohol

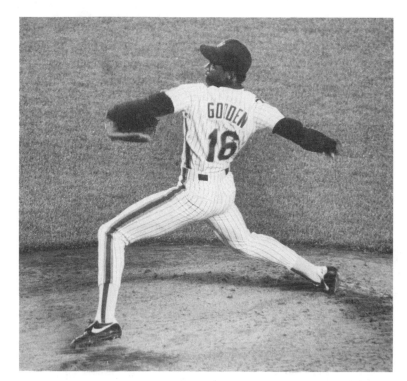

Dwight Gooden of the New York Mets was suspended from baseball when his drug and alcohol problem surfaced.

and at the Betty Ford Center for cocaine. By 1995, both had been suspended from baseball.

Alcohol has been described as a gateway drug. People like Strawberry and Gooden who start with alcohol tend to find themselves also using other drugs. Most young people who use drugs started with alcohol and then moved on to drugs such as marijuana.

Marijuana

Researchers at the University of Michigan found that in the 1993–94 school year, 33 percent of high school seniors and 13 percent of eighth graders smoked marijuana at least once. The numbers showed an increase from the preceding year.

At the college level, marijuana use is declining among student athletes, but just over 24 percent of the respondents to the NCAA drug study still used marijuana in 1993. Almost 60 percent said they started smoking in high school, and 15 percent smoked their first joint in junior high.

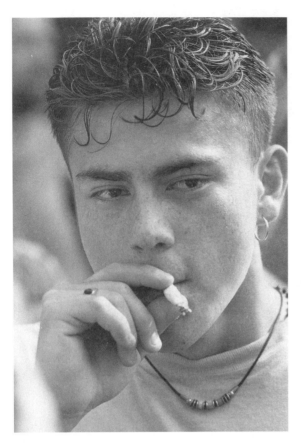

Marijuana consumption is on the rise among young people, according to a 1993–94 study of high schoolers.

Jennifer Capriati was the age of a high school senior when she was arrested for marijuana possession in 1994. Four years earlier she had been called the "Can't-Miss Kid." In 1990, when she beat Martina Navratilova at Wimbledon at the age of fifteen, she was the twenty-sixth highest paid athlete in the world.

"She's the most hyped tennis player of all time," says Pam Shriver, a longtime veteran of the tennis tour. "Nobody can operate with those kinds of expectations without repercussions."

Athletes like Capriati who have used marijuana likely will see a drop in their sports performance. They will feel unsteady and weaker; they may lose steadiness in their hands; and they will have a slower reaction time. Chronic abusers may have memory loss, perhaps feeling less motivated and generally dull.

Marijuana brings the same risks as smoking cigarettes. The chemicals that are trapped in the lungs of a marijuana smoker are just as harmful as those found in tobacco smoke.

Nicotine

Concerned about cigarette smoke, many athletes think it is healthier to use snuff or chewing tobacco than cigarettes. But they are wrong. These products also contain nicotine, and nicotine in any form harms the body.

In *Dying to Win*, Asken reports on an Oklahoma track star:

> He reportedly started using smokeless tobacco at the age of 11 or 12 because he saw his sports heroes using it. He died at

19 from a cancer that had spread from his tongue to his neck. It was his doctor's opinion that the smokeless tobacco has caused his cancer and subsequent death.

In spite of its potential harm, tobacco is not banned by any sports organization. The NCAA, however, conducts nonpunitive tests for nicotine for research purposes. It found that the use of smokeless tobacco is increasing among college athletes. Most often used by males who play baseball and football, smokeless tobacco is now used by male tennis players and track-and-field athletes. Women in tennis, basketball, diving and swimming, and track and field also were using more smokeless tobacco.

Smokeless tobacco

"Contrary to some myths, using smokeless tobacco doesn't improve [sports] performance," say Martha Harding and Kevin Ringhofer. These authors point out in their

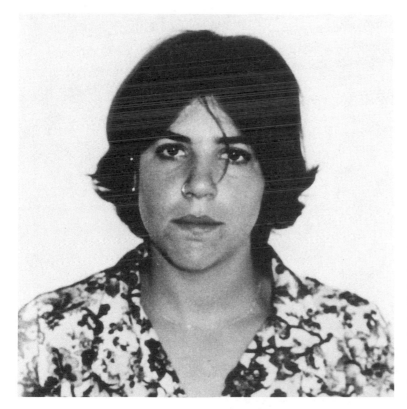

The mug shot taken of Jennifer Capriati after her arrest for marijuana possession in 1994. For athletes like Capriati, who soared to fame in 1990, recreational drugs may relieve the stress of competition.

booklet "The Spitting Image: Is Chewing Tobacco a Part of the Game?" that smokeless tobacco products can negatively affect an athlete's stamina by increasing blood pressure and heart rate. Athletes who swallow tobacco juice can become dizzy or nauseated.

Chewing or dipping can irritate the gums, lips, throat, and stomach. And it can lead to cancer in these areas. Users also experience mood swings. According to "The Spitting Image," "Chewers and dippers can get a buzz from using smokeless tobacco. When the buzz wears off, they feel let down and want to use again. If they are in a situation where they can't use, they can get anxious."

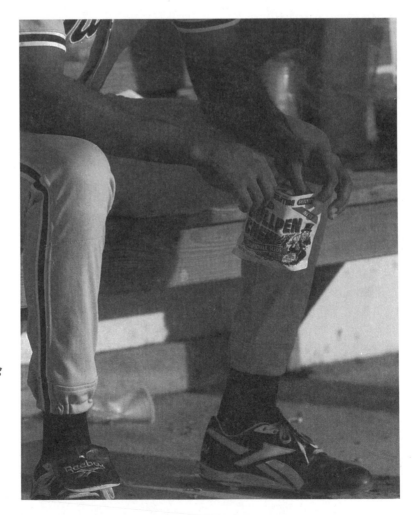

Baseball players have traditionally been heavy users of chewing tobacco despite the drug's side effects. As an alternative to chewing tobacco, this baseball player dips into a tobacco-like pouch of sunflower seeds.

Most athletes get hooked on social drugs because they have relied on these substances as a way to calm their anxiousness. Most began using the drugs as a way to relax and have fun, but those who become addicted find it impossible to kick back and have a normal life. None of these athletes went looking for the grief that comes with drug addictions—damaged health, trouble with the law, loss of a job, or hurtful headlines. But many find one or all of these. What they do not find after abusing alcohol, cocaine, marijuana, or nicotine is the combination of skills and conditioning that will make them better athletes.

5

Drug Testing

MANY ATHLETES WHO use illegal drugs do not want to stop using illegal drugs. They want the competitive edge that comes from steroids and other PAAs, and often they have the support of their trainers. Sports federations and professional organizations worldwide know that many participating athletes use drugs. They conduct tests to find and punish those who do.

Testing begins

Testing for the use of illegal drugs has been in place since before many of today's top athletes were born. Responding to a growing concern about drug abuse, the International Olympic Committee Medical Commission was begun in 1967 to help stop drug abuse.

But the commission knew that making rules was only the first step: it could not control drug use unless it had ways to find and punish those who broke the rules. Drug testing first appeared at the Olympics in 1968 at the Summer Games in Mexico City and at that year's Winter Games in Grenoble, France. But extensive testing did not start until the 1972 Games in Munich.

The IOC commission set out to do what sports organizations at many levels have been trying to do ever since. It named the drugs that foster unfair competition or harm an athlete's health and prohibited their use. It listed these banned drugs, and it set up testing procedures.

Testing methods

Drug-using athletes and their trainers try to be one jump ahead of the testers. When a test succeeds in picking up one type of chemical, athletes look for substances that are not as easy to detect, or for which testing procedures have not been developed. For example, many athletes switched to anabolic steroids when the tests for amphetamine-based stimulants were seen to be effective.

As tests are improved to permit detection of more forms of synthetic steroids, athletes turn to other drugs or to "designer" drugs—drugs that work like steroids but are specially formulated to evade most current testing methods. Ben Johnson's coach, for instance, admitted that Johnson had passed seventeen drug tests in 1986 and 1987, even though he was taking a type of synthetic steroid during this time.

Some drugs elude the testers because they are similar to the body's own chemicals. Testosterone and human growth hormone, for example, are normally present in the

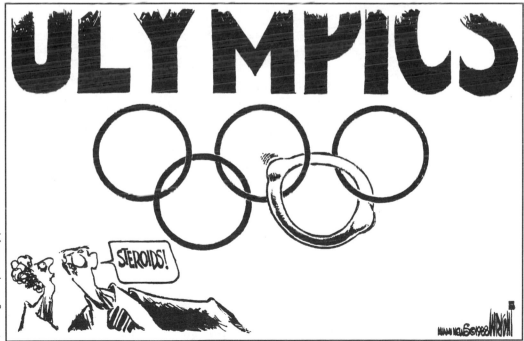

Don Wright. Reprinted by permission: Tribune Media Services.

body. Tests cannot discern by quality alone whether the urine being tested contains an athlete's natural hormones or illegally ingested substances.

Urine tests

Urine tests have been used for more than twenty-five years to detect the presence of steroids, amphetamines, cocaine, marijuana, and alcohol in an athlete's system. Urine tests are becoming more and more accurate and sensitive. Most urine tests usually can detect drugs used up to thirty-six hours before sample collection. One large testing laboratory at University of California at Los Angeles says its tests are sensitive enough to detect a spoonful of sugar dropped into an Olympic-sized swimming pool.

In fall 1995, the U.S. Food and Drug Administration approved the first sweat patch to test for illegal drug use. Applied to the skin, the device gives a reading that indicates the presence of amphetamines, cocaine, and other drugs. About the size of a playing card, the patch is waterproof and can be worn on the back, upper arm, or chest. The patch is also tamperproof: that is, athletes cannot take it off to use drugs and put it back on when they think the drugs have left their bodies. The patch remains active for up to seven days after application.

Fair tests

Most athletes favor fair tests, whether by urinalysis or patch testing, especially at the Olympics, where the sports ideal is stressed. The IOC sets the Olympic testing procedures. It even picks the type of container to be used for the urine tests, selects the labs that will do the work, and decides how the samples will be conveyed from the arenas to the labs.

According to IOC rules, the top four athletes in each singles event are routinely tested, and random tests are conducted for those in heats and finals. During testing, each athlete must be observed urinating into a cup, to ensure that a given specimen really came from the athlete who claims to have produced it. The sample is divided

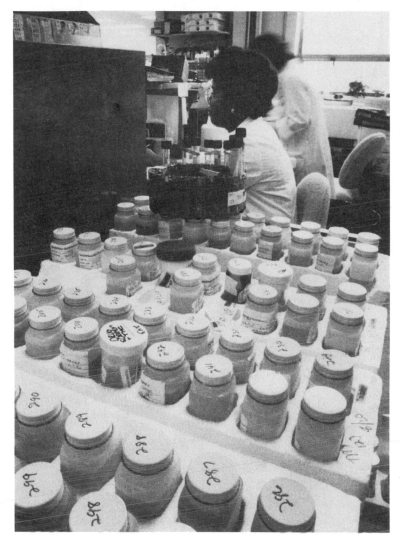

Technicians at the SmithKline Bio-Science Laboratories in Pennsylvania test urine samples for the presence of drugs. Whether athletes should be tested for drugs is a hotly debated topic.

into two cups— A and B—and if the test results from these samples do not agree, the athlete would be retested and an investigation probably would result.

The testing lab works only on coded samples; no athlete's identity is known to the technicians or data analysts. Control samples—samples produced by noncompetitors and deliberately spiked with drugs—are routinely included among the athletes' urine specimens. Thus if a lab fails to report any positive results, the IOC will know that it has a problem.

Robert Voy and his assistant demonstrate the drug testing methods used on Olympic athletes.

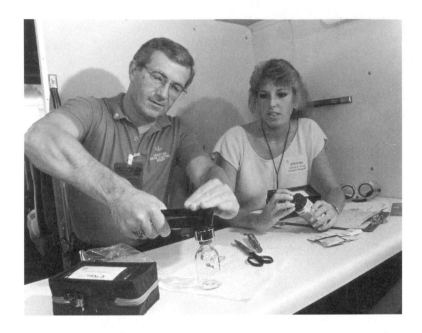

Most likely many more athletes use drugs than are caught in drug tests. In 1984 the chief medical officer for the U.S. Olympic Committee, Robert Voy, conducted a no-penalty test for drugs. That is, athletes who tested positive for drugs were not punished or otherwise penalized. Voy's tests showed that 20 to 50 percent of potential U.S. Olympic athletes were using drugs. But in official tests only about 2 to 3 percent of athletes tested positive for drugs during competitions. The difference in these numbers indicates that athletes have learned how to beat the tests.

Beating the tests

How do athletes beat the tests? There are several ways. For example, they can use drugs the tests cannot detect or they can time their drug use. Since athletes and drug-savvy coaches know how long it takes most chemicals to pass through the human body, it is possible to determine when a competitor needs to stop using a drug to be able to pass the test. Another approach relies on the use of diuretics—drugs that increase the amount of urine the body passes, thus cutting down on the time needed to clear drugs from the system.

Some athletes have gone to the extreme measures of putting someone else's drug-free urine into their bladders before undergoing a urine test. Because the body is always producing urine, clean urine and the athlete's own urine quickly mix in the bladder.

This trick, however, was tried in 1988 by three Canadian weight lifters—Paramjit Gill, David Bolduc, and Jacques Demers, the silver medal winner in 1984. All had been on a steroid program before the 1988 Olympics in Seoul. They intended to beat the tests by stopping their drug use two weeks before departing for South Korea.

The Canadian Weightlifting Federation caught the athletes off guard when it called for tests before the team left Canada. In a panic, the three allowed themselves to be injected with clean urine, but the painful procedure did not work. They failed their tests and were banned from the competition. Many athletes, however, still try this procedure to avoid detection.

A lab technician prepares urine samples taken from athletes participating in the 1988 Olympics. Because drug testing allows officials to eliminate drug users from competition, some athletes go to extreme measures to escape detection.

Masking agents

Some athletes beat the tests by using other drugs that mask or confuse the test results. The antibiotic Probenecid, for example, is a banned substance because it masks the presence of other drugs in the body. In 1992 nationally ranked marathon runner Gordon Bakoulis tested positive for Probenecid after running the New York City Marathon. She received a four-year suspension and returned her winnings from the race.

Bakoulis had taken Probenecid not as a masking agent, but as much-needed therapy for an infection from Lyme disease. Recalling the months when she battled to reverse her suspension, she agreed

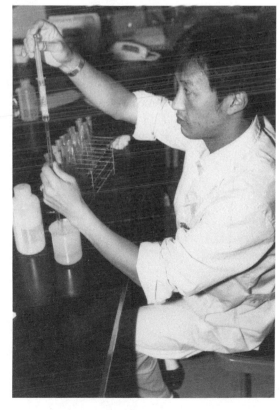

that she should have told her doctor, "I'm an elite runner and subject to drug testing. I can't take certain drugs. Any drug you prescribe I'll need to check with the U.S. Olympic Committee Drug Hotline." But in 1992 she had been focused on only one thing—getting well.

The lawyer from USA Track and Field, the regulating agency for U.S. runners, told Bakoulis she had no case. "'Rules are rules,' he said. There was no question at all that I had broken the rules and therefore should be punished accordingly."

At first the runner resigned herself to the decision. Then, when she read that Ben Johnson had been banned for life for his second drug offense, "the injustice of my suspension hit me like the blow of a sledgehammer. Johnson had cheated; I'd made a mistake. Yet our sport had tarred us both with the same brush."

With the help of a lawyer, Bakoulis got her suspension lifted. Looking back, she says she is not angry. "I believe everyone did what he or she felt was best for the sport, given the current system. But clearly, it's a system that needs some work."

Some claim innocence

Some athletes think the testing system needs work because it blames them even when they did not know their coaches or doctors were giving them illegal pills and injections. Sports officials rarely believe these denials. Most assume that athletes will lie rather than admit to illegal drug use that would remove them from competition. Initially, for example, Johnson insisted that he had never "knowingly" taken steroids. But weeks later a tape recording made by his doctor captured Johnson talking openly about his steroid use.

In fall 1995, U.S. swimmer Jessica Foschi insisted that she had never taken illegal drugs. But she tested positive for anabolic steroids—the first U.S. swimmer to flunk a drug test since 1988. Foschi suggested that someone had spiked her Gatorade, and she passed a lie detector test.

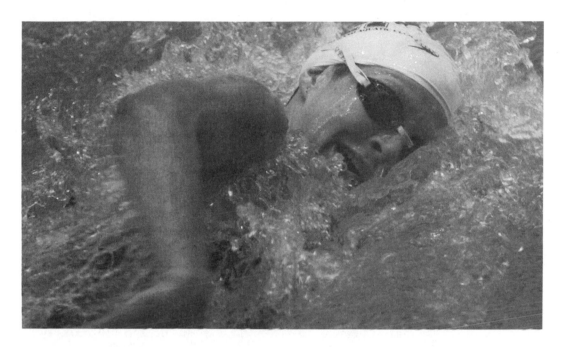

In an unusual turn, the sport's governing body did not suspend Foschi. Instead, a review panel for U.S. Swimming gave her a two-year probation. The ruling enabled her to keep swimming competitively, and even to try out for the 1996 Summer Olympics. As it was, fifteen-year-old Foschi did not swim strongly enough in March 1996 to make the U.S. Olympic swim team.

In 1995, swimmer Jessica Foschi found herself at the center of a controversy when she tested positive for steroids. Foschi insisted that she had never used drugs and suggested that possibly her Gatorade had been spiked with the drug.

Corrupt testing

The Foschi case gives fuel to the argument advanced by some that sports testing is corrupt, unfair, inconsistent, and governed more by politics and favoritism than ethics. Kevin Giles, a track-and-field coach for Australia's teams, told a senate committee in Australia that sometimes even the testers try to help athletes avoid the tests:

> [T]aking Australian teams and other teams from around the world through Europe to the major meetings . . . I would very often be asked by the meet director or one of his aides, "Are all the members of your group okay for drugs testing? Would you mind submitting to drug-testing?" . . . It was obvious that if you said, "We do not want to be tested; they will be found positive" they would not test you.

Discouragement

In an interview for a story on athletes and discouragement, reporter Vicky Rabinowicz quotes one athlete who chose to remain anonymous:

> [D]eals are cut all the time with the [sports] federation and national governing bodies. The big-gun athletes—the world record holders and the medalists—get passed over in the drug testing, so that no scandals take place. That's why I was shocked when Ben Johnson got caught.

Athletes, writes Rabinowicz, are discouraged by the widespread use of AAS, HGH, and other performance-enhancing drugs and methods. Some, she says, suggest two Olympics, one for drug users and one for those who stay clean. Clearly, many of the athletes Rabinowicz interviewed assume that most Olympic-class athletes would fail fair drug tests.

As a way to make the tests fairer and more likely to catch cheaters, sports organizations now conduct unannounced tests of top athletes. The computer program used by the U.S. track federation randomly picks top-ranked

Jackie Joyner-Kersee leads the pack over the hurdles during the 1992 Olympics. Because she ranks as one of the top women athletes, Joyner-Kersee was subjected to several unannounced drug tests in 1991.

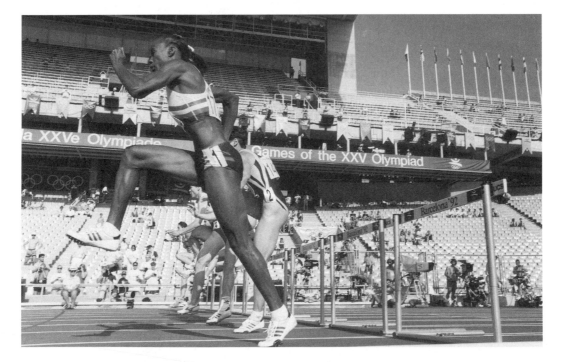

athletes for urine tests throughout the season. In 1991 Jackie Joyner-Kersee, Olympic gold medalist in the long jump and the pentathlon, ranked among the top fifteen competitors in five different events—the high jump, the 200 meters, and the high hurdles, plus her gold medal events. Her success prompted the computer to pull her up for testing three straight weeks and four times during a six-week period.

Bob Kersee, the athlete's husband and coach, called the testing a nuisance. "But the good thing about it is that when the season is over and Jackie sets world records, the last thing we should have to answer are drug-testing questions."

Maybe too tough

Executives for the 1996 Summer Games in Atlanta feared they would have to answer to those who thought the tests were too tough. Some Olympic administrators worried that their top stars would test positive. In 1995 highly sensitive detection machinery led to seventy-seven positive drug tests in weight lifting alone, including a dozen at the prestigious world championships.

A story released by the French newspaper *L'Equipe* said that Russian Olympic Committee president Vitaly Smirnow feared that too many positive tests involving Russian weight lifters would cause the Russian government to reduce its financial support to the Olympics.

Testing in the pros

Testing is done not only in Olympic and Olympic-related events. It also occurs in professional and collegiate sports. Since the late 1960s, amateur and professional sports organizations worldwide have set up drug guidelines.

When the National Basketball Association and the National Basketball Players Association began their Anti-Drug Program in 1983, they included strong provisions for testing. They also stated the penalties for failing to pass the drug tests.

The NBA/NBPA program includes two types of testing. Rookies—those new to professional basketball—are given

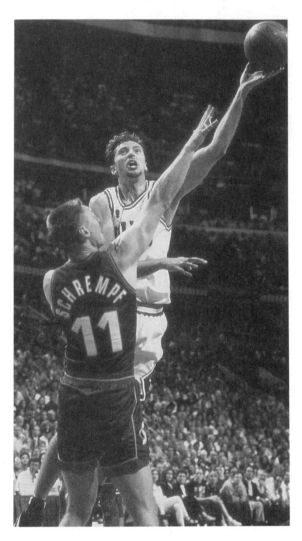

The NBA is among the organizations that have implemented drug testing programs to keep their players drug free.

a urine test once during training camp. A rookie who fails the test is suspended without pay for at least one year. If he satisfactorily completes a drug treatment program, he can return after the year, but he will have to take three more unannounced urine tests during the regular season.

"All players," says the policy, "are also subject to reasonable cause testing—that is, testing based on the player's behavior or other evidence establishing reasonable cause to believe that the player is using a prohibited substance."

If a player behaves in a manner that raises suspicions, or if a team learns of a player's possible drug use, the NBA likely will randomly test for drug use four times during a six-week period without giving the player advance notice.

Any NBA player who is convicted of using heroin or cocaine or pleads guilty to using, possessing, or distributing these drugs is dismissed from the league. A player is also immediately dismissed if drug tests show that he used heroin or cocaine. Dismissed players may reapply to the league after two years.

In the National Football League, players must start the season drug free. The league also uses random testing to catch drug users during the season. In 1989 the Chicago Bears suspended defensive back Maurice Douglass, and the Los Angeles Rams suspended tight end Vernon Kirk. Eleven other NFL players were suspended for using steroids.

Testing in college

Like the professional leagues, the National Collegiate Athletic Association has a detailed testing policy. Any athlete who wants to compete in NCAA sports signs a form giving his or her consent to testing.

"This consent statement," says the NCAA, "is required of all student-athletes." Athletes who do not complete and sign the statement each year cannot compete.

In its 1993 drug survey, the NCAA learned that 33 percent of the athletes surveyed had undergone testing by the NCAA or their respective schools. About 10 percent of those tested said their schools' tests were "easy to beat," and almost 20 percent said that either they or one of their teammates had "beaten" a school-administered drug test.

Testing in high school

Drug tests also occur in some high schools. Since 1990 every athlete takes part in the drug-testing program at Homewood-Flossmoor High School, just south of Chicago. A visiting nurse picks a sample group of students, who then take a urine test. After two positive tests, the young person must enter a counseling and drug treatment program.

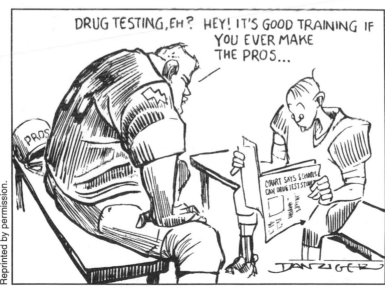

In Sheridan, Indiana, students who play on the Marion-Adams High School teams also have been tested since 1990. The school began the program after a mother found two vials of steroids in her son's gym bag. The school spends about $4,000 a year on drug tests. Sue Kresak, the 1991 president of the Marion-Adams Education Association, said, "I'm afraid that if we stop testing our athletes, they may stop saying 'no' to drugs."

Testing challenges

Some people want to say "no" to drug testing. Sports already has too many rules, some argue. Others believe that testing is an invasion of privacy and violates the right to freedom from unreasonable searches. Others, who point out that testers can make mistakes, go on to conclude that ruined careers will result.

Those who advocate drug testing, especially in schools, found support in a 1995 U.S. Supreme Court decision. The Court ruled six to three that random drug testing in schools does not violate the Fourth Amendment prohibiting unreasonable searches.

The case involved James Acton, an Oregon seventh grader, who in the fall of 1991 signed up to play football. He was cut from the school's team when his parents refused to sign the consent forms allowing drug testing.

Justice Antonin Scalia, who wrote the majority opinion, said the Court looked at three factors when deciding in favor of the tests. First, athletes give up a certain amount of privacy when they agree to undress together in a sports locker room and when they agree to follow a tough athletic schedule. Second, the means for gathering the urine was not intrusive or punishing. Finally, the testing was in line with the great need of the schools to protect children from drugs.

Justice Sandra Day O'Connor, who wrote the dissenting opinion, said the random tests would force millions of youth to undergo "intrusive" urine tests even when they have not given school officials any reason to suspect them of using illegal drugs.

Those in the sports world, however, know that more than suspicion is behind charges of drug abuse. Many hope that the testing programs in professional and amateur sports will curb those suspicions and send a strong message: drugs will not be tolerated.

Testing certainly does not stop suspicions or cheating, but it does reduce illegal behavior. Tests deter some who might otherwise use drugs and ruin their health in the process. Testing also helps restore some people's faith in the overall fairness of sports competitions. Finally, testing procedures put athletes on notice: if you cheat to win, you may get caught, and then you will lose it all.

6

Ethics and Education

"THE DOPING PROBLEM is a crisis in values," say international athletes and educators Saxon White and Ronald Laura. The ethical dilemma—what is right and what is wrong—about drugs and sports focuses on what people are willing to do to win. It also examines whether what they do is unfair to others or harmful to themselves and to sports. This dilemma involves much more than just what athletes think and do about drug use.

These ethical decisions also must be made by coaches and trainers and by people in professional and amateur sports organizations. They must be made, as well, by those who direct sports in countries where athletes' medals are used to build national prestige.

Coaches and trainers

Coaches and trainers sometimes are seen as major obstacles to drug-free sports. Steroids and other performance-enhancing drugs have been handed out in locker rooms. From high schools to the pros, coaches have been known to look away rather than confront an athlete suspected of using drugs.

Many opposed to drugs in sports have called for bans, supplemented by punishments for those who are not tough on drugs, those who actively encourage athletes to use drugs, and those who act as though drugs are all right. Sebastian Coe, the Olympic gold medalist from Britain in the 1,500-meter run in 1980 and 1984, called for more than just a "life ban of offending athletes; we call for the life ban of coaches and the so-called doctors who administer this evil."

Questions about looking the other way or condoning drug use were leveled at the coaches at the University of Miami. Warren Sapp, a 285-pound lineman, had tested positive for drugs seven times while on Miami's team, yet he missed only two games in three years. The University of Miami's drug policy states that after a second positive test, a player is suspended for one game. A third failed test and a player is suspended for the season. Some wondered how Sapp could have tested positive for drugs seven times and still play college ball.

It is a violation of NCAA rules for a school not to follow its own drug policy. Why did Warren Sapp's coaches and school neither punish him nor help him when they had the chance? Why did they look the other way? The answer

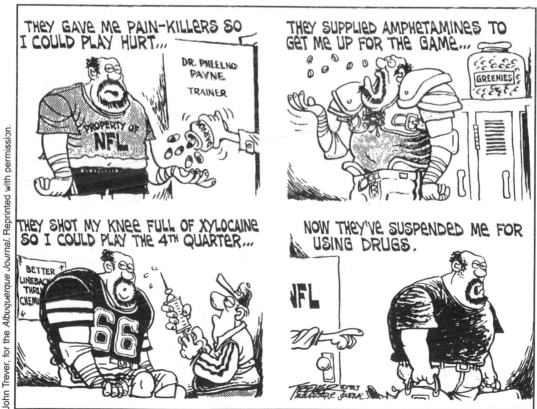

might be that Miami's sports people wanted Sapp to win for Miami more than they wanted Sapp to win for himself.

Rewarding problem athletes

Sportswriter Mark Starr wonders why pro teams continue to hire troublemakers or players addicted to drugs and alcohol and then make them millionaires with hefty contracts. New York Yankees owner George Steinbrenner signed Darryl Strawberry to a $850,000 contract. In spite of a record of drug abuse going back to the mid-1980s, Strawberry has not been off a major league payroll for more than two months. The contract with the Yankees came one week after Strawberry's suspension for cocaine

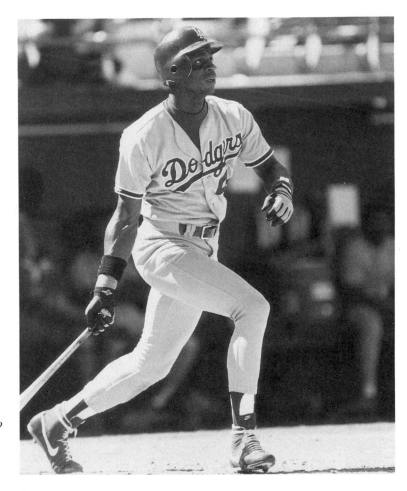

Darryl Strawberry sends the ball flying out of the stadium during the 1991 baseball season. Many people wonder why pro teams continue to hire Strawberry, who has a history of drug abuse.

use had expired and not long after a period of house arrest for tax evasion had been completed.

"He now resumes his career without hitting bottom," Starr writes, "often a key step on the road to recovery. . . . The Yankees may be doing a disservice to Strawberry, whose drug use has cost him jobs with both the Dodgers and the Giants in the past 13 months."

Help from the pros

The National Basketball Association has both help and penalties built into its drug policy. Moreover, education and rehabilitation are included in the Anti-Drug Program begun by the NBA and the National Basketball Players Association in 1983.

Under the NBA's program, a player who voluntarily comes forward to seek drug treatment for cocaine or heroin is given counseling and medical help during and after treatment. Players who admit to drug use for the first time and enter treatment are paid during their treatment. They are not penalized as long as they stay with their drug program. They can be asked to comply with a program of unannounced drug testing following treatment.

Players who voluntarily come forward a second time for help with drugs lose their pay during the treatment time, but they suffer no other penalties. Any player who continues to have problems with drugs after a second treatment program is dismissed from the NBA. The player can apply for reinstatement after two years. The NBA's drug policy covers only cocaine and heroin, but other substances can be added if the NBA and the players' group agree.

The National Football League also has changed its locker-room drug policies with a view to protecting players from addictions and drug abuse. In May 1996, Green Bay Packers quarterback Brett Favre announced that he was entering the NFL's substance abuse program. Favre's father told the media that his son was addicted to painkillers and alcohol.

In a sports story for the *Kansas City Star*, reporter Kent Pulliam wrote, "It hasn't been revealed where Favre got

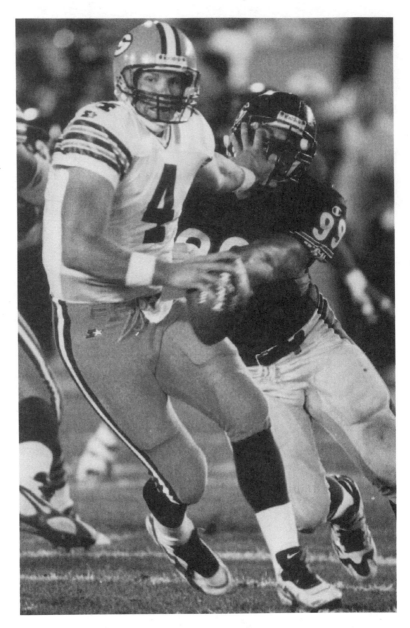

Green Bay Packers quarterback Brett Favre eludes an opponent in this 1995 photo. In May 1996, Favre announced that he was entering the NFL's substance abuse program for treatment of an addiction to pain-killers and alcohol.

the [painkillers], but the days of uppers, downers, or even aspirin—let alone prescription medications—being readily available in NFL locker rooms are gone."

Teams must now record the distribution of all drugs and report such activity to the league. At the Kansas City Chiefs, players sign an agreement not to accept prescription drugs from outside sources. In addition, they all tell their trainers when they take any over-the-counter drugs during the season.

NBA star helps addicted athletes

A major push for drug intervention and prevention is coming not only from teams and leagues, but also from athletes who have experienced drug or alcohol abuse. Former NBA star John Lucas has been clean and sober since he was fired from the Houston Rockets in 1986. When he left the treatment center, he founded the John H. Lucas Enterprise in Houston, a firm specializing in drug and alcohol education, treatment, and rehabilitation. He bought the Miami Tropics, a minor league basketball team, which he used as a way to help athletes stay clean and sober. Six of the ten men on the players' roster were in recovery. The Tropics program included drug therapy sessions and drug testing. In 1992, with Lucas as coach, the Tropics won the U.S. Basketball League Championship

John Lucas rallies his players during a January 1996 game. Lucas, who fought his own battle against drug abuse, has helped other athletes beat their addictions.

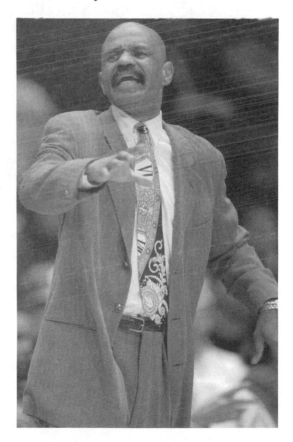

Lucas has worked with dozens of recovering athletes, including the most celebrated San Antonio Spur, NBA All-Star George "the Iceman" Gervin. Lucas says he wants to be a symbol of sobriety for athletes and for fans. He believes his true calling is helping people in recovery.

Other athletes who are recovering addicts and alcoholics also are working with school kids and with other addicted athletes. Former NFL coach Sam Rutigliano started the Inner Circle, a weekly drug counseling and support group for former football players. All-Pro football player Carl Eller now works with the NFL's drug prevention program and with Triumph Life, a private counseling and treatment center in Minneapolis. Eller also helps young people to become drug-free leaders through the United States Athletes Association.

Nations must also help

People trying to clean up drugs in sports know the problem goes well beyond professional-level sports. In the worldwide athletic community, some nations still have a way to go in acknowledging and resolving their drug problems. A sincere effort to stop illegal drug use would include stiff penalties imposed on athletes who test positive for illegal drugs. In Olympic-level competitions, some nations stress the importance of winning to the point of casting doubt on their ethics.

In China today, as in Eastern Europe before the collapse of the Soviet Union, athletes start training at early ages in government-sponsored sports programs that feature rigorous grooming to be winners. Some think this grooming includes drugs.

Olympic-class swimmer Liu Limin was only seven when she left her family to live at a state-run boarding school for athletes. As she trained in China for the 1996 Summer Games in Atlanta, she could read a sign urging the athletes to win for China. "Undergo self-imposed hardship so as to strengthen resolve to wipe out national humiliation," the sign said.

The sign referred to China's humiliation at the 1994 Asian Games where eleven Chinese athletes, including seven swimmers, failed their drug tests. Because she passed her tests and could still compete, Liu felt great pressure to succeed for China. "My only thought was that I had to swim well. . . . If we get many [medals], we can prove again that China is strong, and that it isn't relying on stimulants to build itself up."

China insists that the athletes who failed their tests made a personal decision to use drugs. But many observers wonder. Coaches, doctors, and trainers are suspected of having supplied drugs to the athletes.

China's highly organized approach to sports resembles the methods seen in the 1980s in countries of the Soviet Union, and especially the former East Germany, which was known for its drug labs and its skill at avoiding detection at drug tests. At the Summer Games in Seoul in 1988, East Germany won a total number of 102 medals, second only to the Soviets, with 132.

Countries get tough

When East and West Germany united in 1989, the reunified nation created one of the world's strictest drug-testing programs. In one training year Germany conducted four thousand spot checks on its athletes. Other countries also are cracking down: Canada, Britain, Australia, New Zealand, Norway, and France have adopted strict drug policies, which they take care to enforce.

Other nations are more lax with their drug programs. Chris Wood, writing for *Maclean's*, wrote in 1992: "The United States, for one, has moved only tentatively toward rigorous drug testing of its Olympic athletes." The regrettable result, he says, is that athletes worldwide still do not believe they have a level playing field.

National drug policies deeply affect athletes' willingness to compete without drugs. These policies also affect the ethical decisions teams and athletes make about drugs. But some observers think citizens may help their countries move away from win-at-all-cost attitudes.

Marjorie Blackhurst, a member of Canada's federal task force on drugs, said she believes that attitudes about drugs changed after the many failed drug tests in Seoul. There is, she says, a greater concern for fairness. "Fair play is one of our most strongly held values," she said, "and Canadians were horrified by what happened in Seoul."

Fair play

The NCAA says, "The use of drugs to enhance athletic performance violates the very principles of fair competition." But what does it mean to be fair? The answers to that question help people shape their values about drugs in sports.

Athletes compete under a wide array of circumstances that are not always equal. Talent, training, and resources vary from athlete to athlete, prompting heated debate about what constitutes fairness in sports.

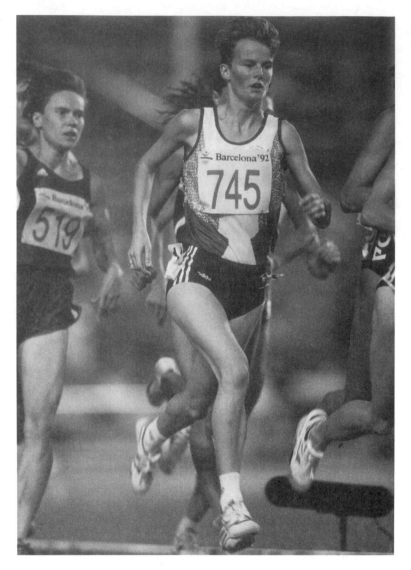

Fair competition, which is the goal, is not the same as equal conditions for all, which cannot be obtained. Talent, luck, and opportunity are not evenly distributed. Similarly, runners wear different shoes, and some shoes are better than others. Some athletes have more money to spend on shoes, and some countries have more money to spend on training runners. These differences are not a matter of fairness.

What is fair and unfair when it comes to drugs? What should be legal and what should be banned? Those who have pondered these questions suggest that drug use is unfair when a healthy athlete takes a drug to gain an unfair advantage in a competition.

This definition makes a distinction between the athlete who takes a cold remedy because he or she is sick and the athlete who takes the drug to have an unfair advantage. Drug use to restore or maintain health is acceptable; drug use that harms health or is accompanied by negative side effects is not.

Some people have suggested that the fair way to handle drugs in sports is for every athlete to be able to use drugs legally. If everyone may use them, then no one has an unfair advantage. But the majority of those concerned about drugs and sports make their decisions about what is fair in large part on what is also healthy. Fairness and health—the combination of those two ideals is what motivates many of the educational programs aimed at keeping athletes safe from drugs. Most of those education programs are directed at young athletes.

Education helps

At the college level, Frank Uryasz, director of sports science at the NCAA, credits educational programs as one factor in the recent decline of drug use, especially steroids, among college athletes. Cocaine use is also down, and many athletes responding to the NCAA survey said they quit using cocaine because they were concerned about their health. Most likely they learned about drug-related health issues from sports programs and coaches.

At the high school level, eight of ten coaches cited in a 1991 Gallup poll of more than a thousand coaches said they considered students' drug and alcohol use to be a "somewhat big" or "very big" problem. About half asked for "special training" so they could better help students who used drugs and alcohol.

The TARGET program also reaches out to high school students. Sponsored by the National Federation of State High School Associations, TARGET wants information about performance and appearance-altering drugs included in all programs aimed at the prevention of use of alcohol and other drugs, in health education, and in athletic programs. "Because PAA drug use is now reported in fifth and sixth graders, these prevention efforts need to begin in early elementary grades," it says.

TARGET also wants to discredit rather than encourage young people who use drugs:

> Athletes who use PAA drugs and attain success receive social approval, admiration for their new body image, and accolades for winning performances as well as scholarships

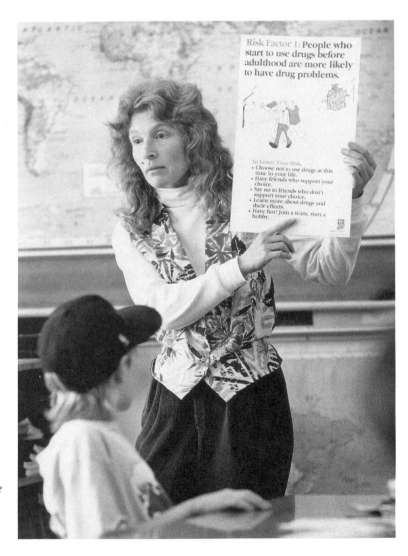

If the war on drugs in sports is to be won, it must begin in the general public. Most people concerned about drug abuse agree that early education is a major weapon in fighting the war.

and other awards. Some acquire worldwide recognition, fame, and fortune, further reinforcing the message that athletes can reap rewards by using PAA drugs.

Athletes who are cared for by their coaches, countries, and team owners and are educated about the harms of drugs will make the right choices about drugs. They will not harm themselves or forsake the ideal of fair competition. International guidelines and regulations must continue to protect them. But the greatest protection must come from within each athlete. For when athletes regulate their own drug behaviors and receive encouragement from others in this effort, fairness and health will be a natural part of sports everywhere.

Glossary

acromegaly: A disorder of the pituitary gland that causes enlargement of hands, feet, and facial features. Nonprescription use of human growth hormones can cause this disorder.

alcohol: A colorless liquid found in beer, wine, and liquor that can cause drunkenness in a person who consumes it.

alcoholism: An illness characterized by excessive drinking and dependence on alcohol. Is often fatal.

amphetamines: Stimulants that increase the heart rate and make the user feel alert and energetic. Often referred to as "speed."

anabolic: Having to do with the building up of muscle.

anabolic androgenic steroids (AAS): Man-made forms of the male hormone testosterone. Taken by injection or in pill form, AAS build muscle mass, power, and speed. They can be harmful to the body.

androgenic: Male-producing. An androgenic hormone, for example, causes masculine changes in the body.

"black market": Describing the illegal business of buying or selling goods, such as drugs, whose sale or use is restricted or controlled by law.

"brake" drugs: Often, hormones used to block or slow down sexual or physical maturation.

caffeine: A stimulant found in coffee, tea, colas, chocolate, and some medications.

clean: Drug free. A clean athlete is one who does not take drugs.

clenbuterol: A chemical used to put more lean meat on cattle. It is used by some athletes to build muscles.

cocaine: An illegal and addictive stimulant drug derived from the coca plant.

corticosteroids: Hormones produced by the adrenal glands that can be used in the treatment of skin allergies, asthma, and joint pain.

crack: A pure form of cocaine that is smoked. Extremely potent, it quickly causes addiction and can be deadly.

diuretics: Drugs that affect the kidneys and cause excessive water loss through the urine. Some athletes use diuretics to lose weight rapidly or to prevent positive testing for drugs.

dope: The general term used for a drug that enhances mental or physical performance in an athletic competition.

estrogen: A female sex hormone.

gland: An organ that produces hormones. The testes are reproductive glands in men, and the ovaries are reproductive glands in women.

heroin: A white, odorless, bitter chemical that is highly addictive.

hormone: A chemical substance made in the body that affects other body functions or processes. For example, some hormones cause facial hair in men, while others cause breasts to grow in women.

human growth hormone (HGH): Made naturally by the body, this hormone stimulates the body to grow and mature. Some athletes illegally use HGH to increase their muscle size and strength.

marijuana: An illegal drug derived from the hemp plant that causes people to feel happy and drowsy. Often referred to as "grass."

nicotine: A highly addictive drug found in tobacco products.

opium: A habit-forming narcotic chemical taken from the juice of unripe poppy seeds.

performance-altering drugs: Drugs taken to improve strength, speed, and physical appearance, such as steroids. Also called performance-enhancing drugs.

pituitary gland: Located at the base of the brain, this organ produces and releases hormones that regulate many body processes such as body growth and reproduction.

progesterone: A female sex hormone.

"roid rage": The violent behavior or feelings of aggression that are caused by the use of anabolic steroids.

stimulants: Drugs such as caffeine and amphetamines that make the user feel alert and wide awake.

strychnine: A poisonous substance that when taken in small amounts can enhance athletic performance.

synthetic: Describing a substance manufactured in a laboratory.

testosterone: A male sex hormone. This hormone causes men to have facial and pubic hair, deep voices, and larger muscles and less body fat than women.

tranquilizers: Drugs taken to make the user feel calm and less nervous.

Organizations to Contact

The following organizations are concerned about alcohol and drug use among athletes, particularly those still in school.

National Clearinghouse for Alcohol and Drug Information (NCADI)
P.O. Box 2345
Rockville, MD 20852
(800) 729-6686

NCADI provides brochures, reports, and a variety of educational materials on drugs. It distributes "Tips for Teens" pamphlets and drug prevention materials.

National Collegiate Athletic Association (NCAA)
6201 College Blvd.
Overland Park, KS 66211-2422
(913) 339-1906

The NCAA works directly with universities, colleges, and athletic associations devoted to intercollegiate athletics. Its Drug Education Committee provides drug education materials and programs to student athletes in elementary- through college-level sports. It also administers programs in education, drug testing, and prevention of the use of alcohol and other drugs.

National Federation of State High School Associations
11724 N.W. Plaza Circle
P.O. Box 20626
Kansas City, MO 64195-0626
(816) 464-5400

The association stimulates and bolsters support for school athletic and spirit programs, as well as activities in music, speech, and debating. As part of its educational mission, the association produces publications and videos on healthy lifestyle issues including information on alcohol, tobacco, steroids, and other drugs.

North American Youth Sport Institute (NAYSI)
4985 Oak Garden Dr.
Kernersville, NC 27284
(910) 784-4926

The institute provides in-service programs, consulting help, and educational materials to agencies, businesses, schools, and organizations that work with youth in sports. It organizes coaches' clinics and workshops for teachers and works with youth sports councils on the topics of fitness, recreation, and sports and health. NAYSI works closely with the organizations American Youth Football and Youth Basketball of America.

U.S. Department of Education
Safe and Drug-Free Schools Program
600 Independence Ave. SW
Room 604 Portals
Washington, DC 20202-6123
(800) 624-0100

The U.S. Department of Education has developed several excellent materials for elementary and high school students. Publications on alcohol, tobacco, drugs, and drug prevention programs are available. They include "Youth and Tobacco," "Youth and Alcohol," and "What Works: Schools Without Drugs."

U.S. Olympic Committee (USOC)
One Olympic Plaza
Colorado Springs, CO 80909

The USOC produces an array of classroom materials, including a magazine, a video, and curriculum guides. Students who want the USOC's free pamphlet for young people should ask for "Inside the Olympic Movement." All requests for the USOC's Drug-Free posters and its drug education videotape must be directed to the Drug Education and Doping Control Program at the USOC.

Women's Sports Foundation
Eisenhower Park
East Meadow, NY 11554
(516) 542-4700

The foundation's goal is to improve the physical, mental, and emotional well-being of women of all ages through sports and fitness. The foundation provides financial support and educational programs for communities, schools, and athletes. Its publications include booklets on drug use and fitness.

Suggestions for Further Reading

Michael J. Asken, *Dying to Win: The Athlete's Guide to Safe and Unsafe Drugs in Sports*. Washington, DC: Acropolis Books, 1988.

Gordon Bakoulis, "Prescription for Disaster," *Runners World*, October 1993.

John Bartimole, "Drugs and the Athlete . . . A Losing Combination," National Collegiate Athletic Association, Overland Park, KS, 1988.

Martin T. Benson, ed., *1995–96 NCAA Drug Education and Drug Testing Programs*. Overland Park, KS: National Collegiate Athletic Association, 1995.

James Deacon, "Biceps in a Bottle," *Maclean's*, May 2, 1994.

Sheryl DeVore, "Big Muscles, Big Problems," *Current Health 2*, November 1990.

Tom Griffin and Roger Svendsen, "Steroids: To Use or Not to Use? A Guide for Students," WBA Ruster Foundation, Sturgis, MI, 1990.

Martha Harding and Kevin Ringhofer, "The Spitting Image: Is Chewing Tobacco a Part of the Game?" National Federation of State High School Associations, Kansas City, MO, April 1994.

Jet, "Use of Illegal Drugs Up Among Youth Across U.S.," January 9, 1995.

Paul Kimmage, "Drugs and Cycling: The Inside Story," *Bicycling*, July 1990.

Jill Liekec, "Image of Hope," *Sports Illustrated*, January 11, 1993.

Steven B. Milburn and Scott R. Smith, "Your Student Athletes Can Help Prevent AOD [Alcohol and Other Drug] Use," *Student Assistance Journal*, November/December 1992.

National Federation of State High School Associations, "Playing Fair, Keeping Fit, Looking Good Without Using Steroids: A Guide to Preventing the Use of Steroids and Other Performance- and Appearance-Altering Drugs," Kansas City, MO, 1992.

Merrell Noden, "A Revealing Inquiry," *Sports Illustrated*, June 5, 1989.

———, "Shot Down," *Sports Illustrated*, March 15, 1993.

Skip Rozin, "Steroids and Sports: What Price Glory?" *Business Week*, October 17, 1994.

Katherine S. Talmadge, *Drugs and Sports*. Frederick, MD: Twenty-first Century Books, 1991.

———, *Focus on Steroids*. Frederick, MD: Twenty-first Century Books, 1991.

Rick Telander, "Mail-Order Muscles," *Sports Illustrated*, November 22, 1993.

Tom Verducci, "The High Price of Hard Living," *Sports Illustrated*, February 27, 1995.

Works Consulted

William A. Anderson, "Second Replication of a National Study of the Substance Use and Abuse Habits of College Student-Athletes," Executive Committee and Drug Education Committee of the National Collegiate Athletic Association, Overland Park, KS, 1993.

Associated Press, "Cowboys' Irvin Is Indicted," *Kansas City Star*, April 2, 1996.

John Ed Bradley, "Pryor Restraint," *Sports Illustrated*, February 13, 1995.

Julie Cart, "They Don't Call It Doping for Nothing," *Women's Sports and Fitness*, November/December 1994.

Chicago Tribune, "Irvin: I Don't Have a Drug Problem," April 10, 1996.

———, "Steelers' Morris Indicted on Drug Charges," March 27, 1996.

Bob Goldman and Ronald Klatz, *Death in the Locker Room II: Drugs & Sports*. Chicago: Elite Sports Medicine Publications, 1992.

Philip Hersh, "Olympic Notebook," *Chicago Tribune*, April 7, 1996.

———, "Panel Drops Sanctions Against Foschi," *Chicago Tribune*, April 9, 1996.

John M. Hoberman and Charles E. Yesalis, "The History of Synthetic Testosterone," *Scientific American*, February 1995.

Jet, "High Court Upholds Random Drug Tests for Athletes," July 17, 1995.

———, "Random Drug Testing Aims at Joyner-Kersee," June 24, 1991.

Ronald S. Laura and Saxon W. White, eds., *Drug Controversy in Sport: The Socio-Ethical and Medical Issues*. North Sydney, Australia: Allen & Unwin, 1991.

D. R. Mottram, ed., *Drugs in Sport*. Champaign, IL: Human Kinetics Books, 1988.

NEA Today, "Debate: Should Student Athletes Be Subject to Random Drug Testing?" May/June 1991.

Craig Neff, "The NFL and Steroids," *Sports Illustrated*, May 22, 1989.

Mary Nemeth and James Deacon, "Scandal: Act 2," *Maclean's*, March 15, 1993.

Newsweek, "Was She Doped or Just Duped?" November 27, 1995.

Kent Pulliam, "NFL Makes It a Pain to Get Prescription Painkillers," *Kansas City Star*, May 16, 1996.

Vicky Rabinowicz, "Athletes and Drugs: A Separate Pace?" *Psychology Today*, July/August 1992.

Mark Starr, "Fault, Miss Capriati," *Maclean's*, May 30, 1994.

———, "One More Time at Bat," *Newsweek*, July 3, 1995.

Dave Toplikar, "Drugs' Downward Spiral," *Lawrence Journal-World*, April 6, 1996.

Robert Voy, *Drugs, Sport, and Politics*. Champaign, IL: Leisure Press, 1991.

Bruce Wallace, "Victory's Cost," *Maclean's*, December 2, 1991.

Alexander Wolff, "Great Fall of China," *Sports Illustrated*, December 19, 1994.

————, "A Real Sapp," *Sports Illustrated*, May 1, 1995.

Chris Wood, "The Perils of Doping," *Maclean's*, July 27, 1992.

Perry A. Zirkel, "Courtside: Drug Test Passes Court Test," *Phi Delta Kappan*, October 1995.

Index

About the Author

Judith Galas has been a reporter and freelance writer for nineteen years and has reported from Montana, New York City, and London. She has a master's degree in journalism from the University of Kansas and makes her home in Lawrence, Kansas.

Picture Credits